Infection, Super Infection and Antimicrobial Management in ICU

Editors

Luca Brazzi
Giorgia Montrucchio

MDPI • Basel • Beijing • Wuhan • Barcelona • Belgrade • Manchester • Tokyo • Cluj • Tianjin

Editors

Luca Brazzi
Department of
Surgical Sciences,
University of Turin,
Turin, Italy

Giorgia Montrucchio
Department of
Surgical Sciences,
University of Turin,
Turin, Italy

Editorial Office
MDPI
St. Alban-Anlage 66
4052 Basel, Switzerland

This is a reprint of articles from the Special Issue published online in the open access journal *Journal of Clinical Medicine* (ISSN 2077-0383) (available at: https://www.mdpi.com/journal/jcm/special_issues/Infection_Super_Infection_Antimicrobial_Management_ICU).

For citation purposes, cite each article independently as indicated on the article page online and as indicated below:

LastName, A.A.; LastName, B.B.; LastName, C.C. Article Title. *Journal Name* **Year**, *Volume Number*, Page Range.

ISBN 978-3-0365-8380-8 (Hbk)
ISBN 978-3-0365-8381-5 (PDF)

Contents

About the Editors

Luca Brazzi

Professor Luca Brazzi is currently a Full Professor of Anesthesia and Intensive Care at the University of Turin (Italy) and Director of Anesthesia and Intensive Care at the University Hospital 'Città della Salute e della Scienza of Turin (Italy)'.

His clinical and scientific activity began in Milan in 1994, where he held the position of Staff Physician at the Ospedale Maggiore Policlinico of Milan and Assistant Professor at the University of Milan.

He was later appointed Associate Professor of Anesthesia and Intensive Care at the University of Sassari (Italy), where he has been Director of Anesthesia and Intensive Care at the University Hospital. He also coordinated the Intensive Care Residency Program of the University of Sassari and, later, of Turin.

His scientific and research activity focuses on acute respiratory failure, extracorporeal respiratory support, and simulation for training.

He has held numerous positions of responsibility in the context of the Italian Society of Anesthesia, Analgesia, Resuscitation and Intensive Care (SIAARTI), as well as in the European Society of Anesthesia and Intensive Care (ESAIC), of which he is currently a member of the Board of Directors.

He is the author of over 200 publications in indexed international journals. His current h-index is 35.

Giorgia Montrucchio

Dr. Giorgia Montrucchio is an Assistant Professor of Anesthesia and Intensive Care at the University of Turin (Italy), and carries out her clinical activity mainly in the Intensive Care Unit of the University Hospital 'Città della Salute e della Scienza' di Turin (Italy).

She is an Infectious Diseases and Anesthesia and Intensive Care specialist, lecturer in the Intensive Care Residency Program, and responsible for degree courses at the University of Turin (Italy).

Her scientific and research activity focuses on infections in critically ill patients, infection and organ damage biomarkers, healthcare-associated infections, antimicrobial multi-resistance, and antimicrobial stewardship.

She collaborates with the European Society of Anesthesia and Intensive Care (ESAIC) as a member of the subforum 'Infection, sepsis and immunology' and with the Italian Society of Anesthesia, Analgesia and Intensive Therapy (SIAARTI) in the context of training and research projects on vascular access in the critically ill patient.

She is the author of over 60 publications in internationally indexed journals, and her current h-index is 13.

Journal of
Clinical Medicine

MDPI

Article

Incidence of Healthcare-Associated Infections in a Neonatal Intensive Care Unit before and during the COVID-19 Pandemic: A Four-Year Retrospective Cohort Study

Mariateresa Ceparano [1], Antonio Sciurti [1], Claudia Isonne [1,*], Valentina Baccolini [1], Giuseppe Migliara [1], Carolina Marzuillo [1], Fabio Natale [2], Gianluca Terrin [2], Paolo Villari [1] and The Collaborating Group †

1 Department of Public Health and Infectious Diseases, Sapienza University of Rome, 00185 Rome, Italy
2 Department of Maternal and Child Health, Policlinico Umberto I, Sapienza University of Rome, 00161 Rome, Italy
* Correspondence: claudia.isonne@uniroma1.it; Tel.: +39-06-49914886
† Collaborators of the Collaborating Group are indicated in the Acknowledgment section.

Abstract: The COVID-19 pandemic may have had an impact on healthcare-associated infection (HAI) rates. In this study, we analyzed the occurrence of HAIs in a neonatal intensive care unit (NICU) of the Umberto I teaching hospital in Rome before and during the pandemic. All infants admitted from 1 March 2018 to 28 February 2022 were included and were divided into four groups according to their admission date: two groups before the pandemic (periods I and II) and two during the pandemic (periods III and IV). The association between risk factors and time-to-first event was analyzed using a multivariable Cox regression model. Over the four-year period, a total of 503 infants were included, and 36 infections were recorded. After adjusting for mechanical ventilation, birth weight, sex, type of delivery, respiratory distress syndrome, and previous use of netilmicin and fluconazole, the multivariable analysis confirmed that being hospitalized during the pandemic periods (III and IV) was the main risk factor for HAI acquisition. Furthermore, a change in the etiology of these infections was observed across the study periods. Together, these findings suggest that patient management during the pandemic was suboptimal and that HAI surveillance protocols should be implemented in the NICU setting promptly.

Keywords: neonatal intensive care unit (NICU); healthcare associated infection (HAI); COVID-19

Citation: Ceparano, M.; Sciurti, A.; Isonne, C.; Baccolini, V.; Migliara, G.; Marzuillo, C.; Natale, F.; Terrin, G.; Villari, P.; The Collaborating Group. Incidence of Healthcare-Associated Infections in a Neonatal Intensive Care Unit before and during the COVID-19 Pandemic: A Four-Year Retrospective Cohort Study. *J. Clin. Med.* **2023**, *12*, 2621. https://doi.org/10.3390/jcm12072621

Academic Editors: Olivier Mimoz, Luca Brazzi and Giorgia Montrucchio

Received: 2 March 2023
Revised: 24 March 2023
Accepted: 29 March 2023
Published: 30 March 2023

1. Introduction

Healthcare-associated infections (HAIs) are among the most serious preventable complications in neonatal intensive care units (NICUs) [1]. Preterm infants are susceptible to HAIs because of their immature immune systems and prolonged need for indwelling catheters [2]; the risk of these diseases is inversely associated with birth weight and gestational age and increases with time spent in care [3]. The most common type of HAI in NICUs is bloodstream infection (BSI), which can occur in isolation or in association with urinary tract infections and meningitis [3]. The main microorganisms responsible for HAIs include *Staphylococcus aureus*, coagulase-negative *Staphylococci*, and *Enterococci*. In addition, recent years have recorded a considerable increase in HAIs sustained by Gram-negative bacteria and fungi, especially *Candida* spp., which are mainly responsible for ventilator-associated pneumonia (VAP) and urinary tract infections, but also for peritonitis and meningitis [3,4].

According to a study conducted in 2016/2017 [5] using the European Centre for Disease Prevention and Control protocol, the prevalence of HAIs in Italian NICUs was around 5%. However, the organizational challenges experienced during the COVID-19 pandemic may have limited the effectiveness of traditional HAI prevention and control efforts, resulting in an increase in their incidence, as already reported for the adult intensive care unit (ICU) of Umberto I teaching hospital of Rome [6] or in a recent systematic review that investigated *Pseudomonas aeruginosa* bacteremia [7]. Indeed, despite NICUs having one of the lowest COVID-related caseloads among all ICUs, they are still vulnerable to indirect adverse effects of the COVID-19 pandemic [8]. During the pandemic, NICUs faced challenges that were different in nature from those in pediatric and adult ICUs; there were particular concerns relating to clinical workflows and parent–child interactions [9,10], including uncertainty in how to address the risk of exposure for mothers and their babies, reorganization of processes and operations aimed at minimizing risks to staff and patients, and frequent changes in clinical scenarios [8].

While the impact of the pandemic on incidence rates of nosocomial infections in adult ICUs has been investigated [6,11–13], data from the NICU setting are scarce. A few indirect effects of the pandemic on NICUs have been described, such as psychological distress or obstacles in implementing family-centered care [14]. In addition, a reduction in hospital-wide availability of alcohol-based hand rubs was reported to be associated with an increase in the rate of central line-associated BSIs in a single-center study [8]. However, few studies have investigated the impact of pandemic-related measures on the incidence of HAIs in preterm infants admitted to NICUs [8,15]. Therefore, the aim of this study was to analyze the occurrence of HAIs in neonates admitted to the NICU of Umberto I teaching hospital of Rome before and during the COVID-19 pandemic and to identify key factors associated with HAI onset.

2. Materials and Methods

2.1. Setting

In this cohort study, we retrospectively analyzed patients hospitalized in the NICU of Umberto I teaching hospital of Rome from 1 March 2018 to 28 February 2022. Patients were followed until discharge or 23 March 2022. The NICU has a total of six beds in which healthcare providers take care of critically ill babies born in this hospital or coming from other hospitals in Rome and the Lazio region via the Neonatal Emergency Transport Service. We followed the STROBE guidelines to report our findings. Microorganisms' antimicrobial susceptibility profiles were defined according to the classification proposed by Magiorakos et al. [16] (if applicable), whereas coagulase-negative *Staphylococci* were considered as susceptible or resistant to oxacillin and/or glycopeptides [17]. The institutional ethics board of the Umberto I teaching hospital of Rome approved this study (protocol no. 888/2022).

2.2. Data Collection

Data about patients hospitalized in the NICU were retrieved from the prospective patient-based HAI surveillance system that has been conducted in the unit since March 2014 by the Department of Public Health and Infectious Diseases of Sapienza University of Rome. The surveillance personnel routinely review and collect data from patients' medical records, including clinical data and microbiological findings, on a weekly basis using a standardized form. All neonates hospitalized in the NICU for at least 48 h are included and followed until their discharge from the NICU. Data on date of birth, date of admission and discharge, sex, gestational age, birth weight (BW), type of delivery, admission diagnosis (preterm birth, twin pregnancy, or respiratory distress syndrome), exposure to invasive devices (days of central line catheterization, including umbilical catheter, central venous catheter and peripherally inserted catheter, and days of mechanical ventilation), use of antimicrobial agents (days), site of infection, date of infection onset, and microorganism isolated are routinely collected. An infection is considered to be healthcare-associated if it occurs 48 h after birth or admission. The surveillance system records central/umbilical line-associated bloodstream infections (CLABSIs) and ventilator-associated pneumonia (VAP) and any other type of infection that occurs during hospitalization, the diagnosis of which is determined by an infectious disease specialist. All infections are defined according to the standard diagnostic criteria published by the Center for Disease Control and Prevention (CDC), adapted to neonatal pathology [18].

2.3. Statistical Analysis

Patients were divided into four groups according to their admission date: period I, from 1 March 2018 to 28 February 2019; period II, from 1 March 2019 to 29 February 2020; period III, from 1 March 2020 to 28 February 2021; and period IV, from 1 March 2021 to 28 February 2022. The date 1 March 2020 was set as the cut-off date between prepandemic and pandemic years. Then, the two preceding and following calendar years were identified for the analysis in order to investigate four equally long time intervals. For each period, descriptive statistics were obtained using means and standard deviations for continuous variables and proportions for dichotomous and categorical variables. For the univariable analysis, the Kruskal–Wallis test was used to compare continuous variables across study periods, whereas Pearson's chi-squared test was used for dichotomous and categorical variables. BW was categorized accord according to the Center for Disease Control/National Healthcare Safety Network (CDC/NHSN) classification [19]. As for exposure to antimicrobial agents, only those used as prophylaxis were considered (i.e., ampicillin, netilmicin, and fluconazole). Use of these antimicrobial agents was coded as (i) dichotomous (yes/no: yes was assigned in the case of having used the antimicrobial agent for at least one day) or (ii) cumulative (sum of the days of antimicrobial use). Similarly, use of devices (i.e., central line and mechanical ventilation) was coded as (i) dichotomous: (yes/no: yes was assigned in the case of having used a device for at least one day) or (ii) cumulative (sum of the days of device use). The in-hospital mortality rate and the HAI incidence rate together with their associated 95% confidence interval (CI) were calculated per 1000 patient days. Because multiple infection events were observed in a few patients, we also estimated the HAI infection rate per 1000 patient days accounting for recurrent events [20].

Time-to-first HAI (i.e., time-to-first CLABSI or VAP) was estimated by survival analysis. Firstly, we estimated the Kaplan–Meier survival function for each period of hospitalization, and survival curves were compared with the log-rank test. Then, the association between period of hospitalization and time-to-first event was assessed through a multivariable Cox regression model for proportional hazard, which provided estimates of the adjusted hazard ratio (aHR) and its associated 95% CI. The main exposure of interest, period of hospitalization, was adjusted for the potential confounders of the association based on expert knowledge [21]. As a result, the final model included the following variables: period of hospitalization (period II was set as the reference category, because it was the period immediately before the pandemic), sex (female vs. male), delivery (spontaneous vs. Cesarean section), birth weight in grams (because no infection was observed in higher BW classes, we used this variable as continuous), respiratory distress syndrome (yes/no), mechanical ventilation use in days (continuous, cumulative exposure in the time period from admission to discharge in patients without HAI or in the time period from admission to the day before HAI onset in patients with HAI), and previous use of netilmicin and fluconazole (yes/no: yes was assigned in the case of having used an antimicrobial agent for at least one day in the time period from admission to discharge in patients without HAI or in the time period from admission to the day before HAI onset in patients with HAI). Interaction terms between the variables were tested considering a p-value < 0.05 as cut-off. The proportionality assumption was checked by testing the statistical significance of interaction terms involving failure time, each one at a time. Multicollinearity was checked using as threshold a variance inflation factor of 5. All analyses were performed using STATA (StataCorp LLC, 4905 Lakeway Drive, College Station, TX, USA), version 17.0. A two-sided p-value < 0.05 was considered statistically significant.

3. Results

3.1. Characteristics of Patients

From 1 March 2018 to 28 February 2022, 564 neonates were hospitalized in the Umberto I teaching hospital of Rome, of which 503 were included in the HAI surveillance system (Table 1). The highest number of admissions occurred in period II with 148 patients, while period III had the lowest (N = 90). Total observation time ranged from 1629 days in period III to 2038 days in period I, with a longer average length of stay in the NICU in period III (18.1 days). A slightly higher proportion of male infants than females was found in periods III and IV, with 52 (57.8%) and 78 (59.1%) infants admitted, respectively, while the gestational age of the infants was similar across the four periods (about 33 weeks). Average BW was similar in periods I, II, and IV (1919.9 g, 2056.1 g, and 2025.7 g, respectively) and slightly lower in period III (1866.6 g). Considering BW classes, the most-represented category was 1501–2500 g, while the least-represented were 750 g or less and 751–1000 g. Regarding the delivery, most infants were born by Cesarean section, a proportion that reached 86.5% in period III. Preterm birth was quite common in all periods (around 80.0%). By contrast, respiratory distress syndrome increased over the years, ranging from 45.1% in period I to 62.9% in period IV, while twin pregnancy occurred less frequently (20–30% of cases).

As for the use of invasive devices, slightly more patients had a central line in periods I and II (69.9% and 64.9%, respectively) compared to periods III and IV (58.9% and 47.0%, respectively), but the average cumulative use in those who had a central line was highest in period III (19.6 days). Similarly, a lower number of patients underwent mechanical ventilation during the pandemic, especially in period IV (9.8%), but the highest average cumulative exposure was observed in period III (14.7 days). Antibacterial consumption was quite high; approximately three out of four patients were administered ampicillin, whereas two out of three were prescribed netilmicin in each period. However, while the cumulative average use of ampicillin was similar throughout the study, the average exposure to netilmicin was reduced in period IV. Fluconazole, on the other hand, was used in a lower proportion of patients (from 6.8% to 16.7%) with the highest average exposure in periods II and III. Lastly, a greater number of deaths were observed in periods I and II, accounting for slightly higher mortality rates (2.5 deaths per 1000 patient days (95% CI: 1.0–5.9) in period I and 3.5 per 1000 patient days (95% CI: 1.7–7.3) in period II).

3.2. Occurrence of HAIs

The prevalence of patients with at least one HAI was greater during the pandemic than prepandemic (3.0% in period I, 3.4% in period II, 11.1% in period III, and 6.8% in period IV), with the highest proportion of patients with at least one CLABSI or VAP in period III (Table 2). A total of four and five HAIs were recorded in periods I and II, respectively, whereas 16 and 11 HAIs were reported in periods III and IV, respectively. The most frequently diagnosed infection was CLABSI in all periods except March 2020–February 2021, in which 50% of infections were VAP. An increase in the incidence rate of HAIs was observed over time, with a peak in period III. After accounting for recurrent HAIs, similar rates were observed.

Differentiating by type of HAI, the CLABSI and VAP incidence rates showed the same trend, with the highest values from March 2020 to February 2021 (Figure 1). However, when we stratified the HAI incidence rates by BW class, we found some differences: the lowest BW classes ($\leq$750 g and 751–1000 g) had the highest rates of HAIs in period IV (Figure 2A), mostly CLABSI (Figure 2B); the middle BW classes (1001–1500 g and 1501–2500 g) showed a small peak in period III (Figure 2A), mainly VAP (Figure 2C) and CLABSI (Figure 2B), respectively. No HAI was diagnosed among patients in the highest BW class (>2500 g) in any period (Figure 2A–C).

Table 1. Key characteristics of the patients admitted to the neonatal intensive care unit of Umberto I teaching hospital of Rome between March 2018 and February 2022 (N = 503) by study period. Results are expressed as number (percentage, %) or mean (standard deviation, SD).

	Period				
	I 1 March 2018 to 28 February 2019	**II** 1 March 2019 to 29 February 2020	**III** 1 March 2020 to 28 February 2021	**IV** 1 March 2021 to 28 February 2022	*p*-Value *
Patients, N	133	148	90	132	
Total observation time, patient days	2038	1999	1629	1925	
Length of NICU stay in days, mean (SD)	15.3 (15.8)	13.5 (15.6)	18.1 (21.7)	14.6 (15.6)	0.470
Sex, N (%)					0.440
Female	61 (45.9)	74 (50.0)	38 (42.2)	54 (40.9)	
Male	72 (54.1)	74 (50.0)	52 (57.8)	78 (59.1)	
Gestational age in weeks, mean (SD) (N = 499)	32.9 (4.3)	33.5 (4.0)	32.8 (4.2)	33.6 (3.7)	0.300
Birth weight in grams, mean (SD)	1919.9 (885.4)	2056.1 (871.6)	1866.6 (881.1)	2025.7 (764.1)	0.180
Birth weight class, N (%)					0.450
≤750 g	7 (5.3)	6 (4.1)	9 (10.0)	8 (6.1)	
751–1000 g	8 (6.0)	8 (5.4)	6 (6.7)	1 (0.8)	
1001–1500 g	32 (24.1)	29 (19.6)	19 (21.1)	27 (20.5)	
1501–2500 g	56 (42.1)	63 (42.6)	36 (40.0)	61 (46.2)	
>2500 g	30 (22.6)	42 (28.4)	20 (22.2)	35 (26.5)	
Delivery, N (%)					0.810
Spontaneous	23 (17.4)	26 (17.8)	12 (13.5)	20 (15.4)	
Cesarean section	109 (82.6)	120 (82.2)	77 (86.5)	110 (84.6)	
Preterm birth, N (%)	105 (78.9)	114 (77.0)	74 (82.2)	106 (80.3)	0.800
Twin pregnancy, N (%)	22 (16.5)	26 (17.6)	25 (27.8)	33 (25.0)	0.094
Respiratory distress syndrome, N (%)	60 (45.1)	79 (53.4)	55 (61.1)	83 (62.9)	0.018
Use of central line, N (%)	93 (69.9)	96 (64.9)	53 (58.9)	62 (47.0)	<0.001
Cumulative days of central line, mean (SD) (N = 304)	11.9 (10.1)	13.3 (16.5)	19.6 (21.4)	13.9 (14.8)	0.350
Use of mechanical ventilation, N (%)	34 (25.6)	38 (25.7)	21 (23.3)	13 (9.8)	0.003
Cumulative days of mechanical ventilation, mean (SD) (N = 106)	7.6 (8.5)	8.6 (15.3)	14.7 (20.4)	10.8 (11.7)	0.370
Use of ampicillin, N (%)	107 (80.5)	116 (78.4)	67 (74.4)	97 (73.5)	0.510
Cumulative days of ampicillin use, mean (SD) (N = 387)	6.9 (2.8)	6.8 (3.1)	6.4 (2.7)	6.0 (2.7)	0.093
Use of netilmicin, N (%)	102 (76.7)	102 (68.9)	61 (67.8)	94 (71.2)	0.420
Cumulative days of netilmicin use, mean (SD) (N = 359)	5.3 (2.2)	5.5 (2.5)	5.8 (2.5)	4.6 (2.3)	<0.001
Use of fluconazole, N (%)	18 (13.5)	14 (9.5)	15 (16.7)	9 (6.8)	0.091
Cumulative days of fluconazole use, mean (SD) (N = 56)	17.3 (12.0)	30.1 (19.5)	34.2 (19.1)	22.2 (16.4)	0.043
NICU deaths, N (%)	5 (3.8)	7 (4.7)	2 (2.2)	4 (3.0)	0.760
NICU mortality, rate × 1000 patient days (95% CI)	2.5 (1.0–5.9)	3.5 (1.7–7.3)	1.2 (0.3–4.9)	2.1 (0.8–5.5)	

NICU: Neonatal Intensive Care Unit. CI: Confidence Interval. HAI: Healthcare-Associated Infection. * Pearson's chi-squared test was used for categorical variables and Kruskal–Wallis test for continuous variables.

Table 2. Key characteristics of healthcare-associated infections (HAIs) diagnosed (N = 36) among patients admitted to the neonatal intensive care unit of Umberto I teaching hospital of Rome between March 2018 and February 2022 (N = 503) by study period. Results are expressed as number (percentage, %) or mean (standard deviation, SD).

	Period				
	I **1 March 2018 to 28 February 2019**	**II** **1 March 2019 to 29 February 2020**	**III** **1 March 2020 to 28 February 2021**	**IV** **1 March 2021 to 28 February 2022**	***p*-Value ***
Patients, N	133	148	90	132	
Patients with at least one HAI, N (%)	4 (3.0)	5 (3.4)	10 (11.1)	9 (6.8)	0.034
Patients with at least one CLABSI, N (%)	4 (3.0)	4 (2.7)	8 (8.9)	8 (6.1)	0.100
Patients with at least one VAP, N (%)	0 (0.0)	1 (0.7)	5 (5.6)	2 (1.5)	0.007
HAIs, N	4	5	16	11	
Type of HAI, N (%)					0.130
CLABSI	4 (100.0)	4 (80.0)	8 (50.0)	9 (81.8)	
VAP	0 (0.0)	1 (20.0)	8 (50.0)	2 (18.2)	
Incidence rate for first HAI × 1000 patient days (95% CI)	2.1 (0.8–5.5)	2.6 (1.1–6.3)	8.4 (4.5–15.6)	5.4 (2.8–10.4)	
Incidence rate for recurrent HAIs × 1000 patient days (95% CI)	2.0 (0.7–5.2)	2.5 (1.0–6.0)	9.4 (5.5–16.0)	5.6 (3.1–10.3)	

CI: Confidence Interval. CLABSI: Central Line-Associated Bloodstream Infection. VAP: Ventilator-Associated Pneumonia. * Pearson's chi-squared test.

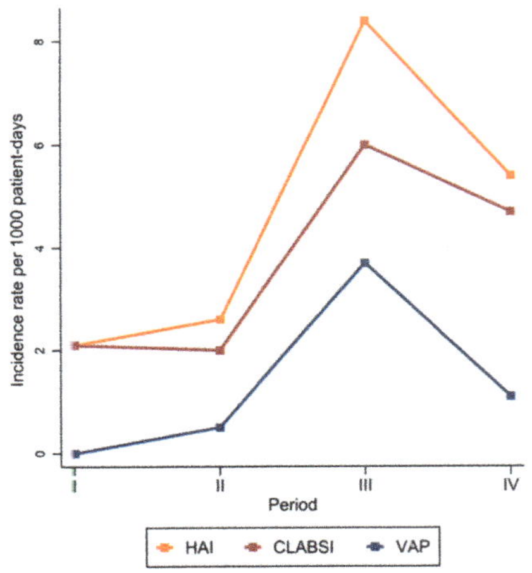

CLABSI: Central Line-Associated Bloodstream Infection. VAP: Ventilator-Associated Pneumonia.

Figure 1. Incidence rate of first healthcare-associated infection (HAI) occurring in patients admitted to the neonatal intensive care unit of Umberto I teaching hospital of Rome between March 2018 and February 2022 by study period.

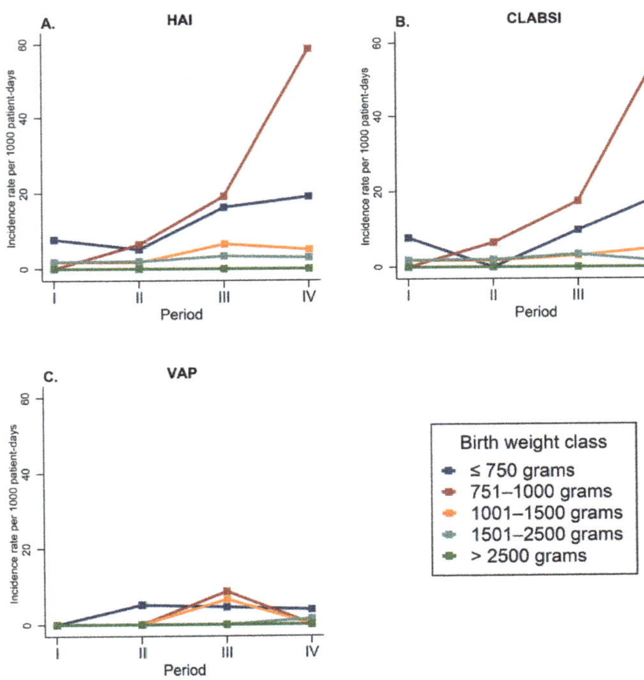

CLABSI: Central Line-Associated Bloodstream Infection. VAP: Ventilator-Associated Pneumonia.

Figure 2. (**A–C**) Incidence rate of first healthcare-associated infection (HAI) occurring in patients admitted to the neonatal intensive care unit of Umberto I teaching hospital of Rome between March 2018 and February 2022 by study period.

The etiology of HAIs across the four study periods varied (Figure 3). *Serratia marcescens* was the pathogen responsible for half the HAIs diagnosed in period I (5.0%), whereas *Klebsiella pneumoniae* was primarily detected in period II (5.0%). By contrast, *Staphylococcus aureus* (22.5%) and coagulase-negative *Staphylococci* (12.5%) were most frequently isolated in period III, as well as in period IV, where infections mainly involved coagulase-negative *Staphylococci* (27.5%), followed by *Escherichia coli* (5.0%). Other microorganisms, such as *Haemophilus influenzae*, were less frequently detected in periods II and III. As for microorganisms' antimicrobial susceptibility patterns, out of 21 pathogens that could be classified according to the Magiorakos criteria [16], no multidrug resistant (MDR) microorganism was isolated in period I, whereas only one MDR isolate was found in period II (4.8%) and period IV (4.8%), respectively. Conversely, the greatest number of MDR microorganisms were isolated in period III (9 microorganisms, 42.9%), alongside an extensively drug-resistant (XDR) microorganism (4.8%). On the other hand, out of the 16 isolates of coagulase-negative *Staphylococci*, the number of such microorganisms resistant to oxacillin increased from 4 in period III (25.0%) to 10 in period IV (62.5%), while only 1 isolate was found to be resistant to both oxacillin and glycopeptides in period IV (6.3%).

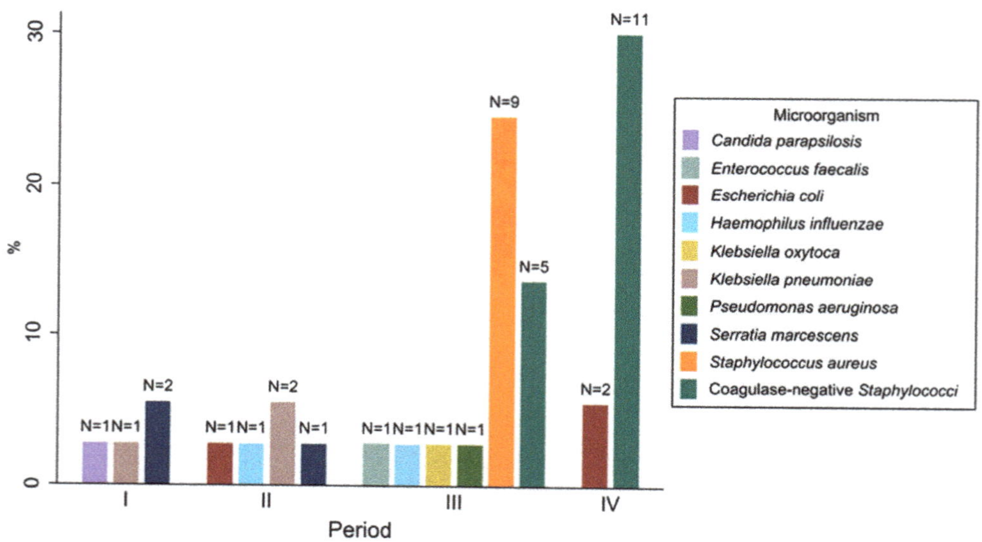

Figure 3. Frequency of isolation of microorganisms (N = 40) responsible for the healthcare-associated infections occurring in patients admitted to the neonatal intensive care unit of Umberto I teaching hospital of Rome between March 2018 and February 2022 by study period.

3.3. *Survival Analysis for First HAI*

Kaplan–Meier estimates for the time of occurrence of the first HAI showed different survival curves across the study periods ($p = 0.042$) (Figure 4). Survival at 30 days decreased from 92.9% (95% CI: 79.3–97.7%) in period I to 82.6% (95% CI: 57.6–93.6%) in period II, and it was further reduced in periods III and IV (60.0%, 95% CI: 35.4–77.8% and 78.3%, 95% CI: 54.4–90.6%, respectively).

A multivariable analysis (Table 3) showed that being hospitalized during the pandemic periods was the main risk factor associated with the contraction of an HAI (period III, aHR: 4.88, 95% CI: 1.33–17.97; period IV, aHR: 6.45, 95% CI: 1.53–27.24). Also, mechanical ventilation (aHR: 1.04, 95% CI: 1.02–1.06) was positively associated with the outcome. By contrast, having a higher BW seemed to be a protective factor against HAIs (aHR: 0.99, 95% CI: 0.98–0.99). Sex, type of delivery, respiratory distress syndrome, and previous use of netilmicin and/or fluconazole did not appear to influence HAI onset.

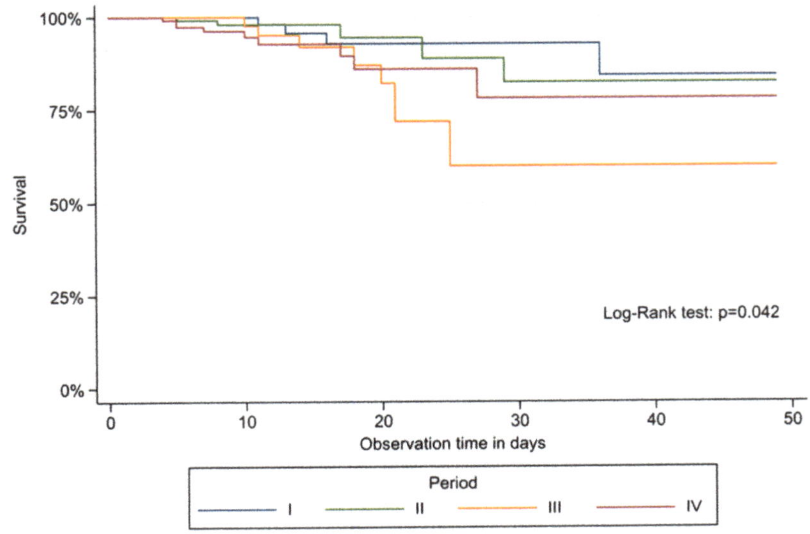

CLABSI: Central Line-Associated Bloodstream Infection. VAP: Ventilator-Associated Pneumonia

Figure 4. Kaplan–Meier survival estimates for time-to-first healthcare-associated infection (HAI) occurring in patients admitted to the neonatal intensive care unit of Umberto I teaching hospital of Rome between March 2018 and February 2022 by study period.

Table 3. Multivariable Cox regression model for first healthcare-associated infection among patients admitted to the neonatal intensive care unit of Umberto I teaching hospital of Rome between March 2018 and February 2022 (N = 503).

	aHR	95% CI	*p*-Value
Period			
II (1 March 2019 to 29 February 2020)	Ref.		
I (1 March 2018 to 28 February 2019)	1.62	0.34–7.67	0.544
III (1 March 2020 to 28 February 2021)	4.88	1.33–17.97	0.017
IV (1 March 2021 to 28 February 2022)	6.45	1.53–27.24	0.011
Sex			
Female	Ref.		
Male	1.08	0.49–2.37	0.843
Delivery			
Spontaneous	Ref.		
Cesarean section	0.73	0.27–1.96	0.537
Birth weight, grams	0.99	0.98–0.99	0.030
Respiratory distress syndrome			
No	Ref.		
Yes	1.86	0.76–4.52	0.172
Mechanical ventilation use, days	1.04	1.02–1.06	<0.001
Previous use of netilmicin			
No	Ref.		
Yes	5.23	0.65–42.40	0.121
Previous use of fluconazole			
No	Ref.		
Yes	0.89	0.33–2.44	0.828

aHR: adjusted Hazard Ratio. CI: Confidence Interval.

4. Discussion

Among the indirect consequences of the COVID-19 pandemic, an increase in the incidence of HAIs has been frequently reported, especially in some wards, such as ICUs [11,22]. However, most studies have focused on adult ICUs, while data on the impact of the pandemic on HAIs in NICUs are still scarce. This is probably because neonates have been less affected by the SARS-CoV-2 infection, and the reorganization of NICUs was less pronounced than in adult ICUs, which needed to cope with a high number of critically ill patients [23]. Among others, starting from March 2020, our NICU limited parent visits as much as possible to avoid overcrowding and reduce the risk of contagion for infants and healthcare personnel. At the same time, the use of personal protective equipment during patient management was mandatorily implemented. In addition, a surveillance protocol based on periodical nasopharyngeal swabs for SARS-CoV-2 detection was established for both parents and healthcare staff. However, in line with the results of Kharrart et al. [8], we recorded an increase in the HAI incidence rate in our NICU during the pandemic, with a peak in the first year (March 2020–February 2021). Therefore, concurrently with the measures taken to control the spread of the virus during the COVID-19 pandemic, it appears that some factors led to less attention being paid to procedures designed to prevent and control traditional HAIs, negatively affecting their incidence. Furthermore, the deficit in individual preventive devices, particularly during the early months of the pandemic, may have increased the fear of infection transmission thereby influencing the implementation of prevention and control measures [24]. Alternatively, or in addition, the increased demand for staff needed to manage COVID-19 patients led hospitals to reorganize their facilities to meet clinical needs [25], and these adaptations may have forced hospitals to hire new healthcare staff, including inexperienced personnel. When this happens in departments such as the NICUs, the shortage of experienced and qualified staff can result in adverse outcomes on newborns, including higher rates of HAIs, as previously documented [26,27]. However, further investigation is needed to determine the specific impact that the discussed factors may have had on HAI acquisition in NICU settings.

As for the HAI type, both CLABSI and VAP rates increased during the pandemic, even though the CLABSI increment was not significant in the univariate analysis, probably due to reduced statistical power. Indeed, despite the lower number of neonates using central lines in these years, the higher average exposure, especially in period III, may at least partially explain the peak in CLABSI incidence recorded between March 2020 and February 2021 [4,28,29]. In addition, period III witnessed a *S. aureus* outbreak in our NICU that accounted for most VAP recorded between May and July 2020. Gram-negative bacteria, particularly *S. marcescens* and *K. pneumoniae*, were the pathogens most frequently responsible for HAIs before the pandemic, in line with data from the literature in which they were often involved in NICU outbreaks [30,31]. In contrast, during the pandemic years, the most frequently detected pathogens were MDR *S. aureus* and oxacillin-resistant coagulase-negative *Staphylococci*, usually the main causes of HAIs in infants [29,32,33]. This change in the microorganism breakdown may help explain why, although more HAIs occurred in periods III and IV, the infant mortality rate did not increase over this time. In fact, the Gram-negative bacteria that circulated in the first two years of surveillance are known to be potentially fatal in NICUs [34–37] compared to the Gram-positive bacteria found in the other two periods, whose infections have recently become more manageable and are less likely to result in patient death [38].

However, our study confirmed that a major risk factor for the occurrence of HAIs in NICUs was low BW [39,40]. This is because such infants are particularly vulnerable to bacterial infections given their immature immune system development, need for prolonged hospitalizations, and need for monitoring, testing, and invasive treatments that circumvent the skin barrier's defense mechanisms [41–44]. This applies to both the lowest BW classes, that accounted for most infections registered throughout the study period, with the highest HAI incidence rates recorded in the 751–1000 g class probably being the result of a smaller number of patients days spent under surveillance compared to the ≤750 g class. Furthermore, while our results show that prolonged mechanical ventilation, which requires the use of breathing circuits known to be important sources and breeding grounds of pathogenic microorganisms [45], contributed to the occurrence of HAIs, variables related to the patients' demographic characteristics and clinical conditions did not influence the outcome. These results partially contrast with those studies in which the male sex and Cesarean section were found to increase HAI occurrence [46,47] but align with findings in which respiratory distress did not show a direct association with HAI onset [47,48]. As for antimicrobials, even though their use did not seem to affect HAI acquisition in our sample, it is worth mentioning that they should be carefully prescribed, because their continued consumption, when inappropriate, can lead to adverse events, including the selection and emergence of highly resistant bacteria [49].

This study has several strengths and limitations. The main strength is the ability to compare data over time. Because data were collected as part of a four-year continuous surveillance system routinely carried out by the Department of Public Health and Infectious Diseases, a potential bias in the results due to overworked NICU staff is unlikely. In addition, to the best of our knowledge, this is one of the few studies that describes and identifies risk factors related to HAI occurrence in a NICU during an emergency period, such as the COVID-19 pandemic. In this regard, we plan to conduct new studies in the near future on the occurrence of HAIs in NICU and ICU settings as the pandemic progresses. In contrast, the first limitation is represented by the fact that we do not have data on the SARS-CoV-2 positivity or negativity status of the infant mothers, even though all hospitalized infants were tested and were SARS-CoV-2 negative. Second, patients discharged from the NICU were no longer under surveillance, although only the most stable patients were chosen for transfer. Third, even though we adjusted for the main risk factors, namely demographic characteristics and use of invasive device and antibiotics, we may have not fully accounted for clinical severity, meaning that some residual confounders may be still present. However, this bias is likely to be constant across time periods. Lastly, we did not study the impact of HAIs on patient mortality, although this was not a goal of our research. Further studies should be conducted to address this issue, together with research that analyzes hand hygiene compliance, which could be of interest to better understand the mechanisms behind any increase or decrease in the incidence rates.

5. Conclusions

We found higher rates of HAIs in our NICU during the COVID-19 pandemic. This, coupled with the fact that the microorganisms involved were different across the study period, suggests a crucial role for patient management and underlines the importance of implementing effective HAI prevention and control strategies [50,51]. Because it is widely recognized that hand hygiene is a highly effective tool in the prevention and control of HAIs [52], it is recommended that further efforts be made to promote adherence to hygiene precautions and increase knowledge and awareness of these issues among NICU healthcare workers.

Author Contributions: Conceptualization, M.C., A.S., and C.I.; methodology, M.C., A.S., C.I., and V.B.; software, A.S. and G.M.; formal analysis, A.S. and G.M.; data curation, M.C., A.S. and Collaborating Group; writing—original draft preparation, M.C., A.S., and C.I.; writing—review and editing, V.B., G.M., C.M., F.N., G.T., and P.V.; visualization, A.S. and M.C.; supervision, P.V.; project administration, C.M. and P.V. All authors have read and agreed to the published version of the manuscript.

Funding: This research received no external funding.

Institutional Review Board Statement: The study was conducted in accordance with the Declaration of Helsinki and approved by Ethics Committee of Sapienza—University of Rome (protocol no. 888/2022 approved on 17 November 2022).

Informed Consent Statement: Patient consent was waived due to being a retrospective observational study that used only data routinely collected during hospitalization.

Data Availability Statement: The data sets generated and analyzed during the current study are available from the corresponding author on reasonable request.

Acknowledgments: The Collaborating Group consists of the following components: Rosa Katia Bellomo, Department of Public Health and Infectious Diseases, Sapienza University of Rome, 00185 Rome, Italy; Vincenzo Cammalleri, Department of Public Health and Infectious Diseases, Sapienza University of Rome, 00185 Rome, Italy; Maria Roberta De Blasiis, Department of Public Health and Infectious Diseases, Sapienza University of Rome, 00185 Rome, Italy; Maria Assunta Donato, Department of Public Health and Infectious Diseases, Sapienza University of Rome, 00185 Rome, Italy; Valentin Imeshtari, Department of Public Health and Infectious Diseases, Sapienza University of Rome, 00185 Rome, Italy; Alessandra Romano, Department of Public Health and Infectious Diseases, Sapienza University of Rome, 00185 Rome, Italy.

Conflicts of Interest: The authors declare no conflict of interest.

References

1. Kumar, S.; Shankar, B.; Arya, S.; Deb, M.; Chellani, H. Healthcare Associated Infections in Neonatal Intensive Care Unit and Its Correlation with Environmental Surveillance. *J. Infect. Public Health* **2018**, *11*, 275–279. [CrossRef]
2. Graham, P.L. Simple Strategies to Reduce Healthcare Associated Infections in the Neonatal Intensive Care Unit: Line, Tube, and Hand Hygiene. *Clin. Perinatol.* **2010**, *37*, 645–653. [CrossRef]
3. Sass, L.; Karlowicz, M.G. Healthcare-Associated Infections in the Neonate. *Princ. Pract. Pediatr. Infect. Dis.* **2018**, 560–566. [CrossRef]
4. Scamardo, M.S.; Dolce, P.; Esposito, E.P.; Raimondi, F.; Triassi, M.; Zarrilli, R. Trends, Risk Factors and Outcomes of Healthcare-Associated Infections in a Neonatal Intensive Care Unit in Italy during 2013–2017. *Ital. J. Pediatr* **2020**, *46*, 34. [CrossRef]
5. Quattrocolo, F.; D'Ambrosio, A.; Corcione, S.; Stillo, M.; Blanco, V.; Gualano, M.; Villa, G.; Voglino, G.; Clemente, S.; Camussi, E.; et al. *Studio di Prevalenza Italiano Sulle Infezioni Correlate All'Assistenza e Sull'uso di Antibiotici Negli Ospedali per Acuti-Protocollo ECDC*; Dipartimento Scienze della Salute Pubblica e Pediatriche, Università di Torino: Turin, Italy, 2018.
6. Baccolini, V.; Migliara, G.; Isonne, C.; Dorelli, B.; Barone, L.C.; Giannini, D.; Marotta, D.; Marte, M.; Mazzalai, E.; Alessandri, F.; et al. The Impact of the COVID-19 Pandemic on Healthcare-Associated Infections in Intensive Care Unit Patients: A Retrospective Cohort Study. *Antimicrob. Resist. Infect. Control.* **2021**, *10*, 87. [CrossRef] [PubMed]
7. Ng, Q.X.; Ong, N.Y.; Lee, D.Y.X.; Yau, C.E.; Lim, Y.L.; Kwa, A.L.H.; Tan, B.H. Trends in *Pseudomonas aeruginosa* (*P. Aeruginosa*) Bacteremia during the COVID-19 Pandemic: A Systematic Review. *Antibiotics* **2023**, *12*, 409. [CrossRef] [PubMed]
8. Kharrat, A.; Neish, A.; Diambomba, Y.; Jain, A. Non-COVID Co-Morbidity: Potential Indirect Consequences of the SARS-CoV-2 Pandemic in a Neonatal Intensive Care Unit. *J. Hosp. Infect.* **2021**, *109*, 65–67. [CrossRef]
9. Griffin, I.; Benarba, F.; Peters, C.; Oyelese, Y.; Murphy, T.; Contreras, D.; Gagliardo, C.; Nwaobasi-Iwuh, E.; Dipentima, M.C.; Schenkman, A. The Impact of COVID-19 Infection on Labor and Delivery, Newborn Nursery, and Neonatal Intensive Care Unit: Prospective Observational Data from a Single Hospital System. *Am. J. Perinatol.* **2020**, *37*, 1022–1030. [CrossRef] [PubMed]
10. Conti, M.G.; Natale, F.; Stolfi, I.; Pedicino, R.; Boscarino, G.; Ajassa, C.; Cardilli, V.; Ciambra, G.L.; Guadalupi, L.; Favata, P.; et al. Consequences of Early Separation of Maternal-Newborn Dyad in Neonates Born to Sars-Cov-2 Positive Mothers: An Observational Study. *Int. J. Environ. Res. Public Health* **2021**, *18*, 5899. [CrossRef]
11. Isonne, C.; Baccolini, V.; Migliara, G.; Ceparano, M.; Alessandri, F.; Ceccarelli, G.; Tellan, G.; Pugliese, F.; de Giusti, M.; de Vito, C.; et al. Comparing the Occurrence of Healthcare-Associated Infections in Patients with and without COVID-19 Hospitalized during the Pandemic: A 16-Month Retrospective Cohort Study in a Hospital Intensive Care Unit. *J. Clin. Med.* **2022**, *11*, 1446. [CrossRef]
12. Ceparano, M.; Baccolini, V.; Migliara, G.; Isonne, C.; Renzi, E.; Tufi, D.; de Vito, C.; de Giusti, M.; Trancassini, M.; Alessandri, F.; et al. Acinetobacter baumannii Isolates from COVID-19 Patients in a Hospital Intensive Care Unit: Molecular Typing and Risk Factors. *Microorganisms* **2022**, *10*, 722. [CrossRef]
13. Deiana, G.; Arghittu, A.; Gentili, D.; Dettori, M.; Palmieri, A.; Masia, M.D.; Azara, A.; Castiglia, P. Impact of the COVID-19 Pandemic on the Prevalence of HAIs and the Use of Antibiotics in an Italian University Hospital. *Healthcare* **2022**, *10*, 1597. [CrossRef] [PubMed]
14. Cena, L.; Biban, P.; Janos, J.; Lavelli, M.; Langfus, J.; Tsai, A.; Youngstrom, E.A.; Stefana, A. The Collateral Impact of COVID-19 Emergency on Neonatal Intensive Care Units and Family-Centered Care: Challenges and Opportunities. *Front. Psychol.* **2021**, *12*, 630594. [CrossRef] [PubMed]
15. Indrio, F.; Salatto, A.; Amato, O.; Bartoli, F.; Capasso, L.; Corvaglia, L.; Maffei, G.; Mosca, F.; Pettoello Mantovani, M.; Raimondi, F.; et al. COVID-19 Pandemic in the Neonatal Intensive Care Unit: Any Effect on Late-Onset Sepsis and Necrotizing Enterocolitis? *Eur. J. Pediatr.* **2022**, *181*, 853–857. [CrossRef]
16. Magiorakos, A.P.; Srinivasan, A.; Carey, R.B.; Carmeli, Y.; Falagas, M.E.; Giske, C.G.; Harbarth, S.; Hindler, J.F.; Kahlmeter, G.; Olsson-Liljequist, B.; et al. Multidrug-Resistant, Extensively Drug-Resistant and Pandrug-Resistant Bacteria: An International Expert Proposal for Interim Standard Definitions for Acquired Resistance. *Clin. Microbiol. Infect.* **2012**, *18*, 268–281. [CrossRef] [PubMed]

17. Becker, K.; Skov, R.L.; von Eiff, C. *Staphylococcus, Micrococcus,* and Other Catalase-Positive Cocci. *Man. Clin. Microbiol.* **2021**, 354–382.
18. Horan, T.C.; Andrus, M.; Dudeck, M.A. CDC/NHSN Surveillance Definition of Health Care-Associated Infection and Criteria for Specific Types of Infections in the Acute Care Setting. *Am. J. Infect. Control.* **2008**, *36*, 309–332. [CrossRef] [PubMed]
19. Centers for Disease Control and Prevention National Healthcare Safety Network (NHSN). *Patient Safety Component Manual;* NHSN: Atlanta, GA, USA, 2023.
20. Prakash Yadav, C. An Overview of Statistical Models for Recurrent Events Analysis: A Review. *Epidemiology* **2018**, *8*, 354. [CrossRef]
21. Talbot, D.; Massamba, V.K. A Descriptive Review of Variable Selection Methods in Four Epidemiologic Journals: There Is Still Room for Improvement. *Eur. J. Epidemiol.* **2019**, *34*, 725–730. [CrossRef] [PubMed]
22. Rosenthal, V.D.; Myatra, S.N.; Divatia, J.V.; Biswas, S.; Shrivastava, A.; Al-Ruzzieh, M.A.; Ayaad, O.; Bat-Erdene, A.; Bat-Erdene, I.; Narankhuu, B.; et al. The Impact of COVID-19 on Health Care–Associated Infections in Intensive Care Units in Low- and Middle-Income Countries: International Nosocomial Infection Control Consortium (INICC) Findings. *Int. J. Infect. Dis.* **2022**, *118*, 83–88. [CrossRef] [PubMed]
23. Shekerdemian, L.S.; Mahmood, N.R.; Wolfe, K.K.; Riggs, B.J.; Ross, C.E.; McKiernan, C.A.; Heidemann, S.M.; Kleinman, L.C.; Sen, A.I.; Hall, M.W.; et al. Characteristics and Outcomes of Children with Coronavirus Disease 2019 (COVID-19) Infection Admitted to US and Canadian Pediatric Intensive Care Units. *JAMA Pediatr.* **2020**, *174*, 868–873. [CrossRef]
24. Thomas Stelfox, H.; Bates, D.W.; Redelmeier, D.A. Safety of Patients Isolated for Infection Control. *JAMA* **2003**, *290*, 1899–1905. [CrossRef] [PubMed]
25. Casafont, C.; Fabrellas, N.; Rivera, P.; Olivé-Ferrer, M.C.; Querol, E.; Venturas, M.; Prats, J.; Cuzco, C.; Frías, C.E.; Pérez-Ortega, S.; et al. Experiences of Nursing Students as Healthcare Aid during the COVID-19 Pandemic in Spain: A Phemonenological Research Study. *Nurse Educ. Today* **2021**, *97*, 104711. [CrossRef] [PubMed]
26. Rogowski, J.A.; Staiger, D.; Patrick, T.; Horbar, J.; Kenny, M.; Lake, E.T. Nurse Staffing and Nicu Infection Rates. *JAMA Pediatr.* **2013**, *167*, 444–450. [CrossRef]
27. Raven, J.H.; Tolhurst, R.J.; Tang, S.; van den Broek, N. What Is Quality in Maternal and Neonatal Health Care? *Midwifery* **2012**, *28*, e676–e683. [CrossRef] [PubMed]
28. Orsi, G.B.; d'Ettorre, G.; Panero, A.; Chiarini, F.; Vullo, V.; Venditti, M. Hospital-Acquired Infection Surveillance in a Neonatal Intensive Care Unit. *Am. J. Infect. Control.* **2009**, *37*, 201–203. [CrossRef] [PubMed]
29. Auriti, C.; Ronchetti, M.P.; Pezzotti, P.; Marrocco, G.; Quondamcarlo, A.; Seganti, G.; Bagnoli, F.; de Felice, C.; Buonocore, G.; Arioni, C.; et al. Determinants of Nosocomial Infection in 6 Neonatal Intensive Care Units: An Italian Multicenter Prospective Cohort Study. *Infect. Control. Hosp. Epidemiol.* **2010**, *31*, 926–933. [CrossRef]
30. Kraus-Haas, M.; Mielke, M.; Simon, A. Update on Outbreaks Reported from Neonatal Intensive Care Units: Serratia Marcescens, Klebsiella Pneumoniae, Acinetobacter baumannii, and *Pseudomonas aeruginosa. Bundesgesundheitsblatt Gesundh. Gesundh.* **2015**, *58*, 308–322. [CrossRef]
31. Morillo, Á.; González, V.; Aguayo, J.; Carreño, C.; Torres, M.J.; Jarana, D.; Artacho, M.J.; Jiménez, F.; Conde, M.; Aznar, J. Brote Epidémico Por Serratia Marcescens En Una Unidad de Cuidados Intensivos Neonatales. *Enferm. Infecc. Microbiol. Clin.* **2016**, *34*, 645–651. [CrossRef]
32. Hocevar, S.N.; Edwards, J.R.; Horan, T.C.; Morrell, G.C.; Iwamoto, M.; Lessa, F.C. Device-Associated Infections among Neonatal Intensive Care Unit Patients: Incidence and Associated Pathogens Reported to the National Healthcare Safety Network, 2006–2008. *Infect. Control. Hosp. Epidemiol.* **2012**, *33*, 1200–1206. [CrossRef]
33. Cailes, B.; Kortsalioudaki, C.; Buttery, J.; Pattnayak, S.; Greenough, A.; Matthes, J.; Bedford Russell, A.; Kennea, N.; Heath, P.T. Epidemiology of UK Neonatal Infections: The NeonIN Infection Surveillance Network. *Arch. Dis. Child Fetal Neonatal. Ed.* **2018**, *103*, F547–F553. [CrossRef]
34. Viswanathan, R.; Singh, A.K.; Mukherjee, S.; Mukherjee, R.; Das, P.; Basu, S. An Outbreak of Neonatal Sepsis Presenting with Exanthematous Rash Caused by Klebsiella Pneumoniae. *Epidemiol. Infect.* **2011**, *139*, 226–228. [CrossRef] [PubMed]
35. Fabbri, G.; Panico, M.; Dallolio, L.; Suzzi, R.; Ciccia, M.; Sandri, F.; Farruggia, P. Outbreak of Ampicillin/Piperacillin-Resistant Klebsiella pneumoniae in a Neonatal Intensive Care Unit (NICU): Investigation and Control Measures. *Int. J. Environ. Res. Public Health* **2013**, *10*, 808–815. [CrossRef]
36. Cristina, M.L.; Sartini, M.; Spagnolo, A.M. Serratia marcescens Infections in Neonatal Intensive Care Units (NICUs). *Int. J. Environ. Res. Public Health* **2019**, *16*, 610. [CrossRef]
37. Yeo, K.T.; Octavia, S.; Lim, K.; Lin, C.; Lin, R.; Thoon, K.C.; Tee, N.W.S.; Yung, C.F. Serratia Marcescens in the Neonatal Intensive Care Unit: A Cluster Investigation Using Molecular Methods. *J. Infect. Public Health* **2020**, *13*, 1006–1011. [CrossRef] [PubMed]
38. Mohzari, Y.; Aljobair, F.; Alrashed, A.; Asdaq, S.M.B.; Alshuraim, R.A.; Asfour, S.S.; Al-Mouqdad, M.M.; Bamogaddam, R.F.; Al-Anazi, D.; Zeilinger, C.E.; et al. Safety and Efficacy of Daptomycin in Neonates with Coagulase-Negative Staphylococci: Case Series Analysis. *Antibiotics* **2021**, *10*, 168. [CrossRef] [PubMed]
39. Polin, R.A.; Denson, S.; Brady, M.T.; Papile, L.A.; Baley, J.E.; Carlo, W.A.; Cummings, J.J.; Kumar, P.; Tan, R.C.; Watterberg, K.L.; et al. Epidemiology and Diagnosis of Health Care—Associated Infections in the NICU. *Pediatrics* **2012**, *129*, e1104–e1109. [CrossRef] [PubMed]
40. Hooven, T.A.; Polin, R.A. Healthcare-Associated Infections in the Hospitalized Neonate: A Review. *Early Hum. Dev.* **2014**, *90*, S4. [CrossRef] [PubMed]

41. Kusari, A.; Han, A.M.; Virgen, C.A.; Matiz, C.; Rasmussen, M.; Friedlander, S.F.; Eichenfield, D.Z. Evidence-Based Skin Care in Preterm Infants. *Pediatr. Dermatol.* **2019**, *36*, 16–23. [CrossRef] [PubMed]
42. Collins, A.; Weitkamp, J.H.; Wynn, J.L. Why Are Preterm Newborns at Increased Risk of Infection? *Arch. Dis. Child Fetal Neonatal. Ed.* **2018**, *103*, F391–F394. [CrossRef]
43. Levy, O. Innate Immunity of the Newborn: Basic Mechanisms and Clinical Correlates. *Nat. Rev. Immunol.* **2007**, *7*, 379–390. [CrossRef]
44. Sampah, M.E.S.; Hackam, D.J. Prenatal Immunity and Influences on Necrotizing Enterocolitis and Associated Neonatal Disorders. *Front. Immunol.* **2021**, *12*, 650709. [CrossRef] [PubMed]
45. Rangelova, V.R.; Raycheva, R.D.; Kevorkyan, A.K.; Krasteva, M.B.; Kalchev, Y.I. Ventilator-Associated Pneumonia in Neonates Admitted to a Tertiary Care NICU in Bulgaria. *Front. Pediatr.* **2022**, *10*, 909217. [CrossRef]
46. Borghesi, A.; Stronati, M. Strategies for the Prevention of Hospital-Acquired Infections in the Neonatal Intensive Care Unit. *J. Hosp. Infect.* **2008**, *68*, 293–300. [CrossRef]
47. Mohammed, D.; el Seifi, O.S. Bacterial Nosocomial Infections in Neonatal Intensive Care Unit, Zagazig University Hospital, Egypt. *Egypt. Pediatr. Assoc. Gaz.* **2014**, *62*, 72–79. [CrossRef]
48. Dal-Bó, K.; Da Silva, R.M.; Sakae, T. Nosocomial Infections in a Neonatal Intensive Care Unit in South Brazil. *Rev. Bras. De Ter. Intensiv.* **2012**, *24*, 381–385. [CrossRef]
49. Tzialla, C.; Borghesi, A.; Serra, G.; Stronati, M.; Corsello, G. Antimicrobial Therapy in Neonatal Intensive Care Unit. *Ital. J. Pediatr.* **2015**, *41*, 27. [CrossRef]
50. Migliara, G.; di Paolo, C.; Barbato, D.; Baccolini, V.; Salerno, C.; Nardi, A.; Alessandri, F.; Giordano, A.; Tufi, D.; Marinelli, L.; et al. Multimodal Surveillance of Healthcare Associated Infections in an Intensive Care Unit of a Large Teaching Hospital. *Ann. Ig* **2019**, *31*, 399–413. [CrossRef]
51. Angelozzi, A.; Caminada, S.; Dorelli, B.; Sindoni, A.; Baccolini, V.; di Paolo, C.; Mele, A.; Salvatori, L.M.; Alessandri, F.; Marzuillo, C.; et al. Knowledge, Attitude, Barriers, Professional Behaviour and Possible Interventions: A Survey on Healthcareassociated Infections among the Healthcare Workers of an Intensive Care Unit in a Large Teaching Hospital in Rome. *Ann. Ig* **2021**, *33*, 628–643. [CrossRef] [PubMed]
52. Allegranzi, B.; Pittet, D. Role of Hand Hygiene in Healthcare-Associated Infection Prevention. *J. Hosp. Infect.* **2009**, *73*, 305–315. [CrossRef] [PubMed]

Journal of
Clinical Medicine

MDPI

Article

Next-Generation Sequencing in Critically Ill COVID-19 Patients with Suspected Bloodstream Infections: A Retrospective Cohort Study

Christoph J. Leitl [1,*], Sandra E. Stoll [1], Wolfgang A. Wetsch [1], Tobias Kammerer [1], Alexander Mathes [1], Bernd W. Böttiger [1], Harald Seifert [2] and Fabian Dusse [1]

1 Department of Anesthesiology and Intensive Care Medicine, Faculty of Medicine, University Hospital of Cologne, University of Cologne, Kerpener Straße 62, 50937 Cologne, Germany
2 Institute for Medical Microbiology, Immunology and Hygiene, Faculty of Medicine, University Hospital of Cologne, University of Cologne, Goldenfelsstraße 19-21, 50935 Cologne, Germany
* Correspondence: christoph.leitl@uk-koeln.de

Abstract: Background: Rapid pathogen identification and appropriate antimicrobial therapy are crucial in critically ill COVID-19 patients with bloodstream infections (BSIs). This study aimed to evaluate the diagnostic performance and potential therapeutic benefit of additional next-generation sequencing (NGS) of microbial DNA from plasma in these patients. Methods: This monocentric descriptive retrospective study reviewed clinical data and pathogen diagnostics in COVID-19 ICU patients. NGS (DISQVER®) and blood culture (BC) samples were obtained on suspicion of BSIs. Data were reviewed regarding the adjustment of antimicrobial therapy and diagnostic procedures seven days after sampling and analyzed using the Chi^2-test. Results: Twenty-five cases with simultaneous NGS and BC sampling were assessed. The NGS positivity rate was 52% (13/25) with the detection of 23 pathogens (14 bacteria, 1 fungus, 8 viruses), and the BC positivity rate was 28% (7/25, 8 bacteria; $p = 0.083$). The NGS-positive patients were older (75 vs. 59.5 years; $p = 0.03$) with a higher prevalence of cardiovascular disease (77% vs. 33%; $p = 0.03$). These NGS results led to diagnostic procedures in four cases and to the commencement of four antimicrobial therapies in three cases. Empirical treatment was considered appropriate and continued in three cases. Conclusions: In COVID-19 patients with suspected BSIs, NGS may provide a higher positivity rate than BC and enable new therapeutic approaches.

Keywords: blood culture; sepsis; antimicrobial therapy; bacteremia; DISQVER®

Citation: Leitl, C.J.; Stoll, S.E.; Wetsch, W.A.; Kammerer, T.; Mathes, A.; Böttiger, B.W.; Seifert, H.; Dusse, F. Next-Generation Sequencing in Critically Ill COVID-19 Patients with Suspected Bloodstream Infections: A Retrospective Cohort Study. *J. Clin. Med.* **2023**, *12*, 1466. https://doi.org/10.3390/jcm12041466

Academic Editors: Timothy E. Albertson and Peter Markus Spieth

Received: 13 January 2023
Revised: 28 January 2023
Accepted: 9 February 2023
Published: 12 February 2023

1. Introduction

Since 2020, the coronavirus disease-2019 (COVID-19) has posed a serious burden on the global healthcare system and especially on intensive care units (ICUs). The progressive availability of vaccines, the emergence of less virulent strains, the growth of clinical experience, and the development of new treatments effectively decreased the number of ICU admissions and overall mortality rates over the course of the pandemic [1–4]. However, in critically ill patients requiring invasive mechanical ventilation, mortality rates remained high throughout the later waves of the pandemic [5,6]. In particular, secondary infections, such as bloodstream infections (BSIs) are strongly associated with poorer outcomes [7–9].

Delayed or inadequate antimicrobial treatment is associated with increased morbidity and mortality rates in sepsis [10–12]. Consequently, the rapid initiation of empiric antimicrobial therapy and the identification of the causative pathogen is crucial.

However, conventional, culture-based methods—which form the current gold-standard for pathogen identification—suffer from limitations, such as delayed results and low test sensitivity, especially with previous exposure to antibiotics [13–15]. Polymerase chain reaction (PCR)-based techniques have been developed as rapid alternatives to culture-based methods, but these approaches often rely on targeted pathogen detection with limited coverages [16].

Recently, next-generation sequencing (NGS)-based methods have emerged as powerful diagnostic platforms for the detection of pathogens in critically ill patients [13,17,18]. The concept of unbiased sequence analysis of circulating cell-free deoxyribonucleic acid (cfDNA) from plasma allows for the identification of bacterial, fungal, and viral microorganisms in one single test, including non-culturable pathogens (e.g., *Tropheryma whipplei* or *Coxiella burnetii*) and irrespective of antimicrobial treatment. In particular, the DISQVER® pathogen test (Noscendo GmbH, Duisburg, Germany) provides comprehensive data analysis and allows differentiation between relevant pathogens and potential microbial contaminants, such as coagulase-negative staphylococci (CNS), by calculating a sepsis-indicating quantifier score [19]. Previous studies have shown a higher sensitivity of NGS-based methods compared to blood cultures (BCs) in patients with suspected sepsis or BSIs, which is potentially beneficial for the optimization of antimicrobial treatments [13,17,18]. However, to date, only a few studies have addressed the clinical impact of complementary NGS diagnostics in patients with either suspected sepsis or BSIs [13,20].

Given the high rate of secondary infections and associated increased mortality in patients with severe COVID-19, we hypothesized that this group in particular would benefit from improved pathogen diagnostics. The aim of this descriptive study was to evaluate the diagnostic performance of NGS-based methods and their potential impact on antimicrobial therapy in a cohort of critically ill COVID-19 patients. To the best of our knowledge, this is the first study investigating the implementation of this new approach in the diagnosis of BSIs in patients with severe COVID-19.

2. Materials and Methods

2.1. Setting and Patients

This retrospective, observational study was conducted between November 2020 and March 2021 at a German 14-bed COVID-19 ICU (Department of Anesthesiology and Intensive Care Medicine, University Hospital of Cologne, Germany). Included in this study were adult patients (age $\geq$ 18 years) with confirmed SARS-CoV-2 infections requiring ICU treatment. A confirmed SARS-CoV-2 infection was defined as a positive reverse transcriptase PCR result obtained from nasopharyngeal swabs and/or lower respiratory tract aspirates. Samples for BC and NGS were obtained when a BSI was suspected by the attending physician based on the clinical signs and symptoms of sepsis. The study was approved by the Ethics Committee of the Medical Faculty of the University of Cologne (Reference No. 21-1444).

2.2. Blood Cultures

Blood samples were obtained either via sterile venipuncture or from a central venous catheter (CVC) after thorough disinfection, according to the institutional standard. At least two pairs of BCs (aerobic and anaerobic, volume 8–10 mL each) were obtained and inoculated (BACTEC, Becton Dickinson, Heidelberg, Germany). The BC bottles were sent to the institutional laboratory and analyzed as previously described [21]. Samples were incubated for up to seven days and the institutional average time to positivity for this method was 13 h.

2.3. Next-Generation Sequencing

Blood samples were drawn under the same conditions as mentioned above, collected into stabilizing blood tubes (Cell-Free DNA BCT CE, Streck, La Vista, NE, USA), and shipped at ambient temperature by a medical logistics service provider to a specialized laboratory (Noscendo GmbH, Reutlingen, Germany). Blood samples were separated to plasma by centrifugation at 1600$\times$ g for 10 min at 4 °C and the plasma supernatant was transferred to a fresh reaction tube. Then, a second centrifugation step at 16,000$\times$ g for 10 min at 4 °C was performed, supernatants were again transferred, and plasma aliquots were further stored. Nucleic acid isolation, quality controls, and library preparation were carried out as previously described [22]. Adequate positive and negative controls accompanied all laboratory and sequencing procedures. All data generated were analyzed using Noscendo's DISQVER® platform, which comprises a curated microbial genome reference database of over 16,000 microbial species, including bacteria, DNA viruses, fungi, and parasites, while potential contaminations and commensals were discriminated from infective agents based on statistical calculations [23]. The analysis time for this method is specified as less than 24 h after the sample is received by the laboratory. Reports were accessible to the treating clinician via an online portal after email notification.

2.4. Virology

Additional diagnostic tests for viruses from blood samples were only conducted if viral DNA was detected by NGS and considered as potentially clinically relevant, or if a viral infection was clinically suspected by the attending physician. The routine virus detection panel for blood samples was performed by real-time PCR, as per institutional protocol, and included herpes simplex virus type 1 and 2 (HSV-1/2), Epstein–Barr virus (EBV), and cytomegalovirus (CMV).

2.5. Data Collection

Data were collected retrospectively through a standardized case report form from electronic and paper medical records. Data included patient demographics, length of ICU and hospital stay, major comorbidities, and discharge data. Clinical data obtained on admission and on the day of sample collection included relevant laboratory data, such as C-reactive protein (CRP), procalcitonin (PCT), and leucocytes, as well as the Sequential Organ Failure Assessment (SOFA) score, therapeutic measures, such as mechanical ventilation, renal replacement therapy, and vasopressor support, antimicrobial treatment, and infectious source control measures. Results from other routine microbiological tests (tracheal secretions, drainage samples, urine, orsamples from surgical sites) were performed within three days, either, before or after blood sample collection for NGS diagnostics were included in the evaluation. Changes in antimicrobial therapy and infectious source control procedures within seven days of NGS sampling were reviewed. Additionally, in patients with viruses detected by NGS, medical records were screened for virological tests and antiviral therapies.

2.6. Data Review

A panel composed of at least two intensivists and one microbiology specialist examined medical files, including clinical parameters, previous course of the disease, consultations with infectious disease specialists, antimicrobial treatments, and results from pathogen diagnostics. Results of the NGS analysis were assessed for clinical relevance and categorized as to whether the results (1) provided any additional or unique findings, (2) led to further diagnostic measures, or (3) affected antimicrobial therapy. The therapeutic impact was further distinguished between (I) initiation of additional antimicrobial treatment, (II) confirmation of therapy already initiated, or (III) discontinuation of ongoing antimicrobial treatment. Identification of typical BC contaminants, such as CNS, was assessed for clinical relevance. Contamination was assumed if the suspected isolates were considered as such, either according to clinical documentation or were present in only one BC and no further action was taken.

2.7. Statistics

Statistical analysis was performed using IBM SPSS statistics software version 28.0 (IBM Corp., Armonk, NY, USA). Continuous data are presented as the median and interquartile range, categorial data are presented as counts and percentages. Quantitative variables were compared using the Mann-Whitney test, qualitative variables were compared using the Chi-square test or Fisher's exact test, as appropriate. A p-value < 0.05 was considered statistically significant.

3. Results

3.1. Study Population

A total of 25 cases with simultaneous BC and NGS sampling were identified for analysis. Demographic data and clinical variables are presented in Table 1. The median (IQR) age was 70 years (56.5–76.5) and patients were predominantly male (16/25, 64%). Patients with positive NGS results were older (75 vs. 59.5 years; $p = 0.03$) and a history of cardiovascular disease was more common in these patients (77% vs. 33%; $p = 0.03$). Other demographical or clinical variables were similar in cases with positive or negative NGS results. The median (IQR) length of ICU stay was 20 days (11–33.5), and in-hospital mortality was 64% (16/25). At the time of sampling, the median (IQR) SOFA score was 8 (6.5–10.5) with 52% of patients (13/25) requiring invasive mechanical ventilation and 88% of patients (22/25) depending on vasopressor support. Antimicrobial therapy was administered in 56% of cases (13/25) and did not significantly affect NGS or BC positivity rates (NGS $p = 0.32$, BC $p = 0.67$). All samples were collected ≥ 48 h after hospital admission.

Table 1. Demographic data and clinical variables at the time of sampling. Demographic and clinical data showed no relevant differences regarding NGS positivity. Data are presented as the median and interquartile range or as counts and percentages, as appropriate. CRP: C-reactive protein; ICU: intensive care unit; IL-6: interleukin 6; NGS: next-generation sequencing; PCT: Procalcitonin; SOFA: sequential organ failure assessment.

Variable	Total (n = 25)	NGS		p
		Positive (n = 13)	Negative (n = 12)	
Age (years)	70.0 (56.5–76.5)	75.0 (70.0–78.5)	59.5 (49.5–71.5)	0.03
Male sex	16 (64)	8 (62)	8 (67)	1
Admission source				
Emergency room	11 (44)	6 (46)	5 (42)	0.82
General hospital ward	7 (28)	4 (31)	4 (33)	0.67
Intermediate care unit	1 (4)	-	1 (8)	0.48
Intensive care unit	6 (24)	3 (23)	2 (17)	0.65
ICU stay (days)	20.0 (11.0–33.5)	22.0 (11.0–44.5)	20.0 (11.3–29.0)	0.61
Mechanical ventilation (days)	13.0 (8.5–27.0)	18.0 (9.0–39.0)	12.0 (4.75–21.3)	0.34
In-hospital death	16 (64)	9 (69)	7 (58)	0.69
Comorbid conditions				
Arterial hypertension	18 (72)	10 (77)	8 (67)	0.67
Cardiovascular disease	14 (56)	10 (77)	4 (33)	0.03
Pulmonary disease	4 (16)	3 (23)	1 (8)	0.59
Renal disease	3 (12)	2 (15)	1 (8)	1
Diabetes mellitus	5 (20)	3 (23)	2 (17)	1
Status at sampling				
SOFA-Score	8.0 (6.5–10.5)	9.00 (6.0–11.5)	7.50 (6.3–8.0)	0.43
Ventilation				
Oxygen support	8 (32)	2 (15)	6 (50)	0.10
Non-invasive ventilation	4 (16)	2 (15)	2 (17)	1
Invasive mechanical ventilation	13 (52)	9 (69)	4 (33)	0.07
Oxygenation (paO_2/FiO_2, mmHg)	144.0 (94.5–183)	144.0 (103–195)	144.0 (87.8–184)	0.74
Vasopressor therapy	22 (88)	12 (92)	10 (83)	0.59
Renal replacement therapy	8 (32)	6 (46)	2 (17)	0.20
Antimicrobial therapy	13 (52)	8 (62)	5 (42)	0.32
Laboratory values				
Leucocytes (10^9/L)	12.4 (8.36–16.5)	12.2 (8.71–18.1)	12.48 (8.27–15.4)	1
Neutrophils (10^9/L)	8.13 (7.20–14.6)	8.13 (7.57–14.8)	9.430 (5.74–13.8)	0.74
Lymphocytes (10^9/L)	0.63 (0.46–1.33)	0.72 (0.48–1.60)	0.62 (0.42–1.09)	0.36
CRP (mg/L)	154 (82.2–219)	130 (66.9–203)	164 (120–252)	0.25
PCT (µg/L)	1.00 (0.40–3.60)	2.20 (0.45–5.45)	0.50 (0.23–1.38)	0.07
IL-6 (ng/L)	82.0 (35.0–686)	109 (35.0–686)	76.0 (34.0–869)	0.87

3.2. NGS and BC Results

Results from 25 NGS tests and 61 sets of BC (minimum of two sets per case) from 25 COVID-19 ICU patients with suspected BSIs were assessed. At least one isolate was detected by NGS or BC in 64% of cases (16/25) and the combination of NGS/BC found 31 microorganisms, including 22 bacteria, 1 fungus, and 8 viruses. An overview of all detected isolates is presented in Table 2.

Table 2. Microorganisms detected by NGS, BC, and PCR. NGS detected 23 isolates (14 bacteria, 1 fungus, and 8 viruses) and provided positive results in 52% (13/25) of cases, whereas BC identified eight bacteria in 28% (7/25) of cases. The most frequently detected bacteria were Enterococcus species in NGS and coagulase-negative staphylococci in BC. Following the identification of viruses by NGS, PCR confirmed four out of five viruses and detected two further isolates of HSV-1. † Coagulase-negative staphylococci. BC: blood culture; HSV-1: herpes simplex virus type 1; NGS: next-generation sequencing; PCR: polymerase chain reaction.

Microorganism	NGS (n = 25)	BC (n = 25)
Bacteria	14	8
Enterococcus faecium	4	1
Escherichia coli	2	1
Enterococcus raffinosus	1	-
Serratia marcescens	1	-
Klebsiella pneumoniae	1	-
Staphylococcus aureus	1	-
Helicobacter pylori	1	-
Bacteroides fragilis	1	-
Staphylococcus epidermidis †	-	1
considered as contaminant		
Staphylococcus epidermidis †	-	3
Corynebacterium imitans	1	-
Xanthomonas campestris	1	-
Staphylococcus hominis †	-	1
Staphylococcus capitis †	-	1
Fungi	1	-
Candida parapsilosis	1	-
	NGS (n = 25)	PCR (n = 4)
Viruses	8	6
Epstein–Barr virus	4	2
Herpes simplex virus type 1	2	4
Cytomegalovirus	2	-

Accounting for all pathogens, NGS showed a statistically non-significant higher positivity rate than BC (NGS: 52%, 13/25 vs. BC: 28%, 7/25; p = 0.083). NGS identified 23 isolates in total (14 bacteria, 1 fungus, and 8 viruses), whereas BC only detected eight bacterial species (p = 0.20).

Contamination of positive samples was less frequent in NGS (15%, 2/13) than in BC (57%, 4/7; p = 0.12). Contaminants found in NGS were *Xanthomonas campestris* (n = 1) and *Corynebacterium imitans* (n = 1), whereas contamination in BC was only caused by CNS (n = 5). These isolates were excluded from the analysis.

The sensitivity for potentially relevant pathogens for NGS and BC combined was 48% (12/25). A comparison of NGS and BC regarding potentially clinically relevant results revealed that NGS provided significantly more positive results than BC (p = 0.01). NGS returned positive results in 48% of cases (12/25) and identified 12 bacteria, 1 fungus, and 8 viruses. Three bacteria considered relevant were detected by BC in 12% of cases (3/25).

3.3. Direct Comparison of NGS and BC

Excluding viruses from NGS results for a more direct comparison, positive results were detected in 36% of cases (9/25) by NGS and in 12% of cases (3/12) by BC (p = 0.05). Both methods returned positive results in three cases and agreed on two bacterial species (*Escherichia coli* and *Enterococcus faecium*). In the remaining specimen, NGS and BC provided inconsistent findings (NGS: *Staphylococcus aureus*, *E. faecium*, *Serratia marcescens*; BC: *Staphylococcus epidermidis*). In nine cases with positive NGS results (seven bacteria, one fungus, and seven viruses), BC analysis remained negative. In 13 cases, no clinically relevant pathogen was found by either method.

3.4. Diagnostic Benefit of NGS

Compared to BC alone, additional NGS diagnostics provided further information in 44% of cases (11/25). NGS identified ten bacteria and one fungus that remained undetected in simultaneously collected BC samples.

Even when including results from other routine microbiological tests, such as surgical swabs, tracheal secretions, and urine, NGS identified four bacteria and one fungus, which were not found in conventional diagnostics (*E. faecium*, n = 2; *Bacteroides fragilis*, n = 1; *Helicobacter pylori*, n = 1; *Candida parapsilosis*, n = 1). NGS confirmed a systemic infection in four cases by detecting six bacteria in the bloodstream, which were otherwise only identified in samples taken directly from the septic focus (abdomen, n = 1, *E. faecium*, *Enterococcus. raffinosus*; lung n = 3, *E. coli*, *S. marcescens*, *S. aureus*, *Klebsiella pneumoniae*).

Since routine screening for viraemia was not routinely performed, NGS revealed eight viral isolates in seven specimens (EBV: n = 4; HSV-1: n = 2; CMV: n = 2), which would otherwise have remained undetected.

3.5. Additional Viral Diagnostic

In four out of seven cases with positive viral NGS, additional PCR confirmed four out of five viruses. EBV and HSV-1 were each confirmed in two out of two cases by PCR. Additionally, HSV-1 was detected by PCR in two further samples, which were missed by NGS. In one patient, positive HSV-1 NGS results led to the suspicion of herpes simplex encephalitis, which was consequently excluded by PCR from cerebrospinal fluid after lumbar puncture.

3.6. Antimicrobial Therapy

Results from additional NGS analysis affected therapy in 20% of all cases (5/25) (Table 3, Figure 1). Identification of clinically relevant pathogens by NGS led to the initiation of four antimicrobial therapies in three cases:

(1) Aciclovir was administered in two patients following positive NGS results for HSV-1, with confirmation by PCR.

(2) Vancomycin treatment was started in two patients after the detection of *E. faecium* by NGS.

Besides clinical factors, NGS further contributed to the continuation of empirical antimicrobial therapy in three cases. Considering the lack of antimicrobial susceptibility testing, empirical antimicrobial treatment was assumed to be appropriate after NGS provided the only identification of causative pathogens in blood samples. NGS did not substantially contribute to the termination of therapy in any of these cases.

Table 3. Contribution of NGS to the optimization of antimicrobial therapy. NGS results led to the initiation of four targeted therapies in three cases. Aciclovir was administered in two cases after HSV-1 was detected by NGS and confirmed by PCR. Vancomycin was started in two cases following the detection of E. faecium by NGS. In three cases, following pathogen detection by NGS, ongoing empiric therapy was considered appropriate and was continued accordingly. BAL: bronchoalveolar lavage; BC: blood culture; EBV: Epstein–Barr virus; HSV-1: herpes simplex virus type 1; NGS: next-generation sequencing; PCR: polymerase chain reaction.

ID	Age/Sex	(Suspected) Source of Infection	Diagnostic Method			Antimicrobial Therapy	
			NGS	BC	Other	Empiric	Contribution of NGS
N3	79/f	Pulmonary	*X. campestris*, HSV-1	Negative	Serum (PCR): HSV-1	Meropenem	Initiation of aciclovir treatment
N8	70/m	Pulmonary	*B. fragilis*, EBV	Negative	Serum (PCR): EBV	Piperacillin/ tazobactam	Confirmation of empiric therapy
N12	78/m	Pulmonary	*E. faecium*, HSV-1, EBV	Negative	Serum (PCR): HSV-1	Meropenem	Initiation of vancomycin and aciclovir treatment
N19	31/m	Unknown	*S. aureus*, *S. marcescens*, *E. faecium*	*S. epidermidis*	BAL: *S. aureus*	Meropenem	Initiation of vancomycin treatment, confirmation of empiric therapy
N25	80/f	Pulmonary or wound	*K. pneumoniae*	Negative	BAL: *K. pneumoniae*	Meropenem	Confirmation of empiric therapy

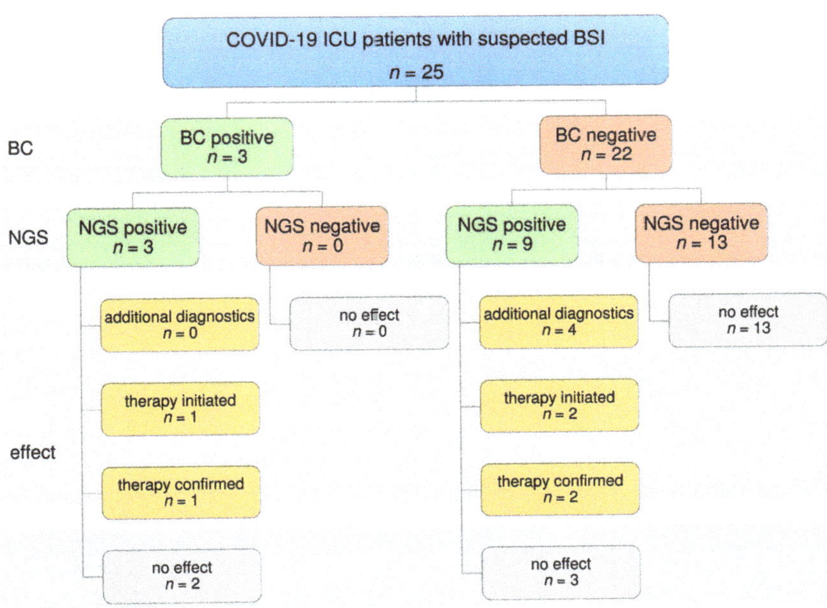

Figure 1. Diagnostic and therapeutic contribution of additional NGS considering BC positivity. BC failed to detect relevant pathogens in 22 of 25 cases. In six of these cases, additional NGS led to further diagnostic tests or contributed to the optimization of antimicrobial therapy. BC: blood culture; BSI: bloodstream infection; NGS: next-generation sequencing.

4. Discussion

This retrospective study investigated the diagnostic performance and potential impact on antimicrobial therapy of additional NGS pathogen diagnostics in COVID-19 ICU patients. NGS was able to detect three times as many bacterial or fungal pathogens in blood samples compared to BC alone ($p = 0.05$). Moreover, NGS detected a viral reactivation in 28% of patients, which would have remained undiscovered by standard diagnostic alone. Based on these results, NGS directly led to the initiation of targeted antimicrobial therapy in 12% of all cases and contributed to the continuation of appropriate therapy in 12% of cases, considering the overall clinical context. NGS led to additional diagnostic procedures, which potentially altered therapy.

In this study, bacterial BSIs were diagnosed by BC analysis in only 12% of cases despite corresponding clinical symptoms. This may be due to the limitations faced by classical culture-based methods: (1) low sensitivity, especially for slow-growing and fastidious organisms, (2) interference due to prior antibiotic exposure, (3) contamination often led to false positive results, and (4) long turnaround time, as standard culture methods typically require 12–36 h for positive signaling and up to 72 h for accurate pathogen identification, including antimicrobial susceptibility testing [13–15].

NGS analysis detected ten additional bacteria as well as one fungus compared to BC in this study cohort. Furthermore, six bacteria were detected in the bloodstream, which otherwise would have been regarded as localized infections (i.e., isolates were only detected in routine non-blood samples). Previous studies reported a 1.5–5.2-fold increase in sensitivity by NGS in patients with suspected sepsis compared to BC [13,17,18]. Our results are in line with these previous studies and demonstrate a higher positivity rate of NGS in the detection of bacteria or fungi compared to BC analysis, in COVID-19 patients (36% vs. 12%, $p = 0.05$).

4.1. *Confirmation of Positive BC Results by NGS*

In only 3 of 25 cases were relevant pathogens detected by both BC and NGS. BC confirmed NGS results in two cases, yet was unable to detect one clinically relevant bacterium in one patient: *S. epidermidis* was isolated in two sets of BCs drawn from a CVC in one patient, whereas NGS detected three different bacteria. These BC results were considered catheter-related BSI according to clinical documentation and, consequently, the CVC was removed, and ongoing antimicrobial treatment continued.

A putative lack of pathogens in NGS analysis might be explained by a technical analysis algorithm. As described in a previous study, isolates might have been identified by NGS but not reported due to a low read count and stringent threshold settings during analysis [13]. Thus, low concentrations of pathogens prevent further analysis and might lead to disagreement between the two methods [24]. Further research will be necessary to address this question and possibly improve analysis algorithms.

4.2. *Defining Antimicrobial Therapy Using NGS*

This study examined the potential impact of NGS results on the choice of antimicrobial treatment. In three cases, four antimicrobial therapies were initiated following positive NGS results. In addition, NGS found pathogens in twelve cases, in which BC remained negative. In three of those cases, empirical therapy was deemed appropriate, and no adjustment seemed necessary. In some cases, the identification of additional pathogens in the bloodstream might have even wider implications, as demonstrated in one case. While conventional methods only found *S. aureus* in respiratory samples and BC remained negative, NGS detected *S. aureus* DNA in the bloodstream. This could have warranted a prolonged duration of antimicrobial therapy and further diagnostic procedures, such as echocardiography to assess for endocarditis. Although this study was not designed to demonstrate a significant benefit of NGS regarding therapy improvement, it can be hypothesized that additional NGS diagnostics may lead to the optimization of antimicrobial therapy in certain critically ill COVID-19 patients. However, given the high cost of NGS compared to standard diagnostics and the still unclear overall limited therapeutic benefit, the indication for the use of NGS should be carefully considered.

4.3. Contamination

An unusually high rate of contamination by CNS in BC diagnostics was observed in this study: CNS were detected in 16% of all specimens and in 57% of positive specimens, which is significantly higher than the usual false-positivity rate reported in our annual pathogen and resistance statistics. In two extensive reviews, performed before SARS-CoV-2 emerged, the overall contamination rates of BC were notably lower and ranged from only 0.6 to 12.5% [25,26]. During the pandemic, a general increase in contamination rate in specimens from COVID-19 individuals was observed, presumably caused by a high workload, newly trained staff, wearing full personal protective equipment, and time pressures [27–30]. Since this study was conducted during the peak of the second and third waves of the pandemic, these aspects may also have been major contributors to this study. In contrast, no CNS were identified in any specimen by NGS. This circumstance may reflect methodological differences. NGS analysis only targets cell-free DNA released by degradation processes or immune system interaction. In cases of contamination, bacterial cells remain mostly intact, avoiding DNA release, which consecutively leads to negative NGS results. This clearly differs from the BC methodology, in which vital bacteria are cultivated followed by positive signaling.

4.4. Value of NGS in the Diagnosis of Fungal Infections

Critically ill COVID-19 patients are at increased risk of developing secondary fungal infections such as COVID-19-associated pulmonary aspergillosis and candidemia [31–36]. In this study, one isolate of *C. parapsilosis* was found only by NGS. However, the result was not considered clinically relevant. According to current guidelines, the diagnosis of candidemia could have warranted additional interventions, such as CVC removal and ophthalmological examination [37]. However, recent studies reported inconsistent results regarding the benefit of NGS in the detection of systemic fungal infections and larger prospective studies will be needed to assess this question [13,17,18,24].

4.5. Value of NGS in the Diagnosis of Viral Infections

Reactivation of latent viruses is common in patients with sepsis and may be even more frequent in patients with severe COVID-19 [38–43]. However, tests for viral infections in clinical routines are lacking. In our study, the implementation of additional NGS analysis led to the identification of 8 viruses in 25 patients, which would have been missed by standard diagnostics. However, in the absence of a clinically apparent viral disease in most cases, the clinical relevance and therapeutic implications of these results remain unclear.

In two patients, treatment with aciclovir was initiated following the identification of HSV-1 by NGS. However, data regarding the prognostic implications of HSV reactivation in patients with COVID-19 is inconclusive, while the only randomized controlled trial on aciclovir treatment in non-COVID-19 patients found no benefit on morbidity or mortality [31,39,40,44,45]. Whether viral reactivation of HSV or CMV in critically ill patients reflects true viral disease (and, therefore, represents possible treatment strategies), or is merely indicative of an immunocompromised state remains controversial and requires further investigation.

4.6. Methodological Characteristics and Limitations of NGS

The relevance of the microorganisms detected by NGS often remains unclear. Clinical experience and treatment recommendations are limited or lacking. Similar to other molecular genetic detection methods, it is uncertain whether the detection of cfDNA corresponds to clinically relevant infection. The genomic material obtained could originate from non-viable or commensal microorganisms and, therefore, might lead to false positive results and mimic an active infection. Furthermore, molecular techniques, currently do not allow for antimicrobial susceptibility testing [16]. In our institution, NGS currently offers no advantage over culture-based diagnostics in terms of turn-around time for logistic reasons. Improved workflows that might provide faster results in the future are currently under investigation [23]. Results of prospective studies showing a positive effect of NGS on clinical outcomes and, thus, justifying the additional costs are still pending [22].

Identifying microorganisms of uncertain clinical relevance and lack of antimicrobial susceptibility testing can result in antimicrobial overtreatment and prevent de-escalation and rational use of antibiotics. These technical limitations demonstrate that NGS-based analysis cannot be used as a substitute for cultural methods, but rather may be considered as a complementary test in patients with severe COVID-19.

4.7. Limitations

This study suffers from numerous limitations, which are mainly attributable to the retrospective study design and the limited cohort. As such, the study design was not suitable to investigate the impact of additional NGS-based diagnostics on morbidity and mortality. A very specific subgroup of patients with severe COVID-19 treated in the ICU was examined, consequently, our results cannot be generalized to other patient groups. The lack of routine screening for common viral infections impedes any direct comparison of the two methods, while sample collection from different sites could lead to divergent results between the methods. Significant differences in demographic variables, such as age or pre-existing diseases, could constitute confounding factors and the small number of individual pathogens precluded an analysis of the association between read count, outcome, and clinical relevance. Despite a comprehensive review of clinical data and documentation, important information may have been unavailable, potentially biasing the evaluation of treatment decisions.

5. Conclusions

The results of our study suggest that NGS-based diagnostics might offer a higher positivity rate than conventional culture-based methods and, therefore, may enable new therapeutic approaches in critically ill COVID-19 patients. However, further experience regarding the interpretation of the results is required and treatment decisions should be carefully considered to avoid overtreatment. Larger, prospective studies will be necessary to determine whether the identification of additional pathogens by NGS can improve the outcome of critically ill ICU patients with severe COVID-19.

Author Contributions: Conceptualization, C.J.L. and F.D.; Investigation, C.J.L., S.E.S., T.K., H.S. and F.D.; Supervision, F.D.; Writing—original draft, C.J.L.; Writing—review & editing, S.E.S., W.A.W., A.M., B.W.B., H.S. and F.D. All authors have read and agreed to the published version of the manuscript.

Funding: We acknowledge support for the Article Processing Charge from the DFG (German Research Foundation, 491454339).

Institutional Review Board Statement: The study was conducted according to the guidelines of the Declaration of Helsinki and approved by the Ethics Committee of the Medical Faculty of the University of Cologne (Reference No. 21-1444).

Informed Consent Statement: Patient consent was waived due to its retrospective design.

Data Availability Statement: The datasets used and analyzed during the current study are available from the corresponding author upon reasonable request.

Acknowledgments: The authors thank Noscendo GmbH for performing the NGS analysis and for providing expertise on general technical inquiries. We also thank Susanna Dreißig and Samuel Steinbach for their help with data collection.

Conflicts of Interest: The authors declare no conflict of interest.

References

1. Asch, D.A.; Sheils, N.E.; Islam, N.; Chen, Y.; Werner, R.M.; Buresh, J.; Doshi, J.A. Variation in US Hospital Mortality Rates for Patients Admitted With COVID-19 During the First 6 Months of the Pandemic. *JAMA Intern. Med.* **2021**, *181*, 471. [CrossRef]
2. Horwitz, L.I.; Jones, S.A.; Cerfolio, R.J.; Francois, F.; Greco, J.; Rudy, B.; Petrilli, C.M. Trends in COVID-19 Risk-Adjusted Mortality Rates. *J. Hosp. Med.* **2020**, *16*, 90–92. [CrossRef]
3. Sigal, A.; Milo, R.; Jassat, W. Estimating disease severity of Omicron and Delta SARS-CoV-2 infections. *Nat. Rev. Immunol.* **2022**, *22*, 267–269. [CrossRef]
4. Anesi, G.L.; Jablonski, D.J.; Harhay, M.O.; Atkins, J.H.; Bajaj, J.; Baston, C.; Brennan, P.J.; Candeloro, C.L.; Catalano, L.M.; Cereda, M.F.; et al. Characteristics, Outcomes, and Trends of Patients with COVID-19–Related Critical Illness at a Learning Health System in the United States. *Ann. Intern. Med.* **2021**, *174*, 613–621. [CrossRef]
5. Karagiannidis, C.; Windisch, W.; McAuley, D.F.; Welte, T.; Busse, R. Major differences in ICU admissions during the first and second COVID-19 wave in Germany. *Lancet Respir. Med.* **2021**, *9*, e47–e48. [CrossRef] [PubMed]
6. Contou, D.; Fraissé, M.; Pajot, O.; Tirolien, J.-A.; Mentec, H.; Plantefève, G. Comparison between first and second wave among critically ill COVID-19 patients admitted to a French ICU: No prognostic improvement during the second wave? *Crit. Care* **2021**, *25*, 1–4. [CrossRef] [PubMed]
7. De Santis, V.; Corona, A.; Vitale, D.; Nencini, C.; Potalivo, A.; Prete, A.; Zani, G.; Malfatto, A.; Tritapepe, L.; Taddei, S.; et al. Bacterial infections in critically ill patients with SARS-2-COVID-19 infection: Results of a prospective observational multicenter study. *Infection* **2021**, *50*, 1–10. [CrossRef]
8. Silva, D.; Lima, C.; Magalhães, V.; Baltazar, L.; Peres, N.; Caligiorne, R.; Moura, A.; Fereguetti, T.; Martins, J.; Rabelo, L.; et al. Fungal and bacterial coinfections increase mortality of severely ill COVID-19 patients. *J. Hosp. Infect.* **2021**, *113*, 145–154. [CrossRef]
9. Shafran, N.; Shafran, I.; Ben-Zvi, H.; Sofer, S.; Sheena, L.; Krause, I.; Shlomai, A.; Goldberg, E.; Sklan, E.H. Secondary bacterial infection in COVID-19 patients is a stronger predictor for death compared to influenza patients. *Sci. Rep.* **2021**, *11*, 1–8. [CrossRef] [PubMed]
10. Ferrer, R.; Martin-Loeches, I.; Phillips, G.; Osborn, T.M.; Townsend, S.; Dellinger, R.P.; Artigas, A.; Schorr, C.; Levy, M.M. Empiric Antibiotic Treatment Reduces Mortality in Severe Sepsis and Septic Shock From the First Hour. *Crit. Care Med.* **2014**, *42*, 1749–1755. [CrossRef] [PubMed]
11. Liu, V.X.; Fielding-Singh, V.; Greene, J.D.; Baker, J.M.; Iwashyna, T.J.; Bhattacharya, J.; Escobar, G.J. The Timing of Early Antibiotics and Hospital Mortality in Sepsis. *Am. J. Respir. Crit. Care Med.* **2017**, *196*, 856–863. [CrossRef]
12. Yokota, P.K.O.; Marra, A.R.; Martino, M.D.V.; Victor, E.S.; Durão, M.S.; Edmond, M.; Dos Santos, O.F.P. Impact of Appropriate Antimicrobial Therapy for Patients with Severe Sepsis and Septic Shock—A Quality Improvement Study. *PLoS ONE* **2014**, *9*, e104475. [CrossRef] [PubMed]
13. Grumaz, S.; Grumaz, C.; Vainshtein, Y.; Stevens, P.; Glanz, K.; Decker, S.O.; Hofer, S.; Weigand, M.A.; Brenner, T.; Sohn, K. Enhanced Performance of Next-Generation Sequencing Diagnostics Compared With Standard of Care Microbiological Diagnostics in Patients Suffering From Septic Shock. *Crit. Care Med.* **2019**, *47*, e394–e402. [CrossRef]
14. Schmitz, R.P.; Keller, P.M.; Baier, M.; Hagel, S.; Pletz, M.W.; Brunkhorst, F.M. Quality of blood culture testing—A survey in intensive care units and microbiological laboratories across four European countries. *Crit. Care* **2013**, *17*, R248. [CrossRef]
15. Vincent, J.-L.; Brealey, D.; Libert, N.; Abidi, N.E.; O'Dwyer, M.; Zacharowski, K.; Mikaszewska-Sokolewicz, M.; Schrenzel, J.; Simon, F.; Wilks, M.; et al. Rapid Diagnosis of Infection in the Critically Ill, a Multicenter Study of Molecular Detection in Bloodstream Infections, Pneumonia, and Sterile Site Infections. *Crit. Care Med.* **2015**, *43*, 2283–2291. [CrossRef] [PubMed]
16. Timsit, J.-F.; Ruppé, E.; Barbier, F.; Tabah, A.; Bassetti, M. Bloodstream infections in critically ill patients: An expert statement. *Intensiv. Care Med.* **2020**, *46*, 266–284. [CrossRef]
17. Long, Y.; Zhang, Y.; Gong, Y.; Sun, R.; Su, L.; Lin, X.; Shen, A.; Zhou, J.; Caiji, Z.; Wang, X.; et al. Diagnosis of Sepsis with Cell-free DNA by Next-Generation Sequencing Technology in ICU Patients. *Arch. Med. Res.* **2016**, *47*, 365–371. [CrossRef] [PubMed]
18. Di Ren, D.; Ren, C.; Yao, R.; Zhang, L.; Liang, X.; Li, G.; Wang, J.; Meng, X.; Liu, J.; Ye, Y.; et al. The microbiological diagnostic performance of metagenomic next-generation sequencing in patients with sepsis. *BMC Infect. Dis.* **2021**, *21*, 1–9. [CrossRef]
19. Grumaz, S.; Stevens, P.; Grumaz, C.; Decker, S.O.; Weigand, M.A.; Hofer, S.; Brenner, T.; von Haeseler, A.; Sohn, K. Next-generation sequencing diagnostics of bacteremia in septic patients. *Genome Med.* **2016**, *8*, 1–13. [CrossRef]
20. Kattner, S.; Herbstreit, F.; Schmidt, K.; Stevens, P.; Grumaz, S.; Dubler, S.; Rath, P.-M.; Brenner, T. Next-Generation Sequencing–Based Decision Support for Intensivists in Difficult-to-Diagnose Disease States: A Case Report of Invasive Cerebral Aspergillosis. *A&A Pr.* **2021**, *15*, e01447. [CrossRef]
21. Ehren, K.; Meißner, A.; Jazmati, N.; Wille, J.; Jung, N.; Vehreschild, J.J.; Hellmich, M.; Seifert, H. Clinical Impact of Rapid Species Identification From Positive Blood Cultures With Same-day Phenotypic Antimicrobial Susceptibility Testing on the Management and Outcome of Bloodstream Infections. *Clin. Infect. Dis.* **2019**, *70*, 1285–1293. [CrossRef]
22. Brenner, T.; Skarabis, A.; Stevens, P.; Axnick, J.; Haug, P.; Grumaz, S.; Bruckner, T.; Luntz, S.; Witzke, O.; Pletz, M.W.; et al. Optimization of sepsis therapy based on patient-specific digital precision diagnostics using next generation sequencing (DigiSep-Trial)—Study protocol for a randomized, controlled, interventional, open-label, multicenter trial. *Trials* **2021**, *22*, 1–12. [CrossRef]

23. Grumaz, C.; Hoffmann, A.; Vainshtein, Y.; Kopp, M.; Grumaz, S.; Stevens, P.; Decker, S.O.; Weigand, M.A.; Hofer, S.; Brenner, T.; et al. Rapid Next-Generation Sequencing–Based Diagnostics of Bacteremia in Septic Patients. *J. Mol. Diagn.* **2020**, *22*, 405–418. [CrossRef]
24. Decker, S.O.; Sigl, A.; Grumaz, C.; Stevens, P.; Vainshtein, Y.; Zimmermann, S.; Weigand, M.A.; Hofer, S.; Sohn, K.; Brenner, T. Immune-Response Patterns and Next Generation Sequencing Diagnostics for the Detection of Mycoses in Patients with Septic Shock—Results of a Combined Clinical and Experimental Investigation. *Int. J. Mol. Sci.* **2017**, *18*, 1796. [CrossRef]
25. Hall, K.K.; Lyman, J.A. Updated Review of Blood Culture Contamination. *Clin. Microbiol. Rev.* **2006**, *19*, 788–802. [CrossRef]
26. Doern, G.V.; Carroll, K.C.; Diekema, D.J.; Garey, K.W.; Rupp, M.E.; Weinstein, M.P.; Sexton, D.J. Practical Guidance for Clinical Microbiology Laboratories: A Comprehensive Update on the Problem of Blood Culture Contamination and a Discussion of Methods for Addressing the Problem. *Clin. Microbiol. Rev.* **2019**, *33*, e00009-19. [CrossRef]
27. Sacchetti, B.; Travis, J.; Steed, L.L.; Webb, G. Effects of COVID-19 on Blood Culture Contamination at a Tertiary Care Academic Medical Center. *Microbiol. Spectr.* **2022**, *10*, e00277-22. [CrossRef]
28. Self, W.H.; Speroff, T.; Grijalva, C.G.; McNaughton, C.D.; Ashburn, J.; Liu, D.; Arbogast, P.G.; Russ, S.; Storrow, A.B.; Talbot, T.R. Reducing Blood Culture Contamination in the Emergency Department: An Interrupted Time Series Quality Improvement Study. *Acad. Emerg. Med.* **2013**, *20*, 89–97. [CrossRef] [PubMed]
29. Russo, E.; Bolondi, G.; Gamberini, E.; Santonastaso, D.P.; Circelli, A.; Spiga, M.; Sambri, V.; Agnoletti, V. Increased blood culture contamination rate during COVID-19 outbreak in intensive care unit: A brief report from a single-centre. *J. Intensiv. Care Soc.* **2021**, *23*, 500–502. [CrossRef] [PubMed]
30. Yu, D.; Ininbergs, K.; Hedman, K.; Giske, C.G.; Strålin, K.; Özenci, V. Low prevalence of bloodstream infection and high blood culture contamination rates in patients with COVID-19. *PLoS ONE* **2020**, *15*, e0242533. [CrossRef] [PubMed]
31. Gangneux, J.-P.; Dannaoui, E.; Fekkar, A.; Luyt, C.-E.; Botterel, F.; De Prost, N.; Tadié, J.-M.; Reizine, F.; Houzé, S.; Timsit, J.-F.; et al. Fungal infections in mechanically ventilated patients with COVID-19 during the first wave: The French multicentre MYCOVID study. *Lancet Respir. Med.* **2021**, *10*, 180–190. [CrossRef]
32. Koehler, P.; Cornely, O.A.; Böttiger, B.W.; Dusse, F.; Eichenauer, D.A.; Fuchs, F.; Hallek, M.; Jung, N.; Klein, F.; Persigehl, T.; et al. COVID-19 associated pulmonary aspergillosis. *Mycoses* **2020**, *63*, 528–534. [CrossRef] [PubMed]
33. Alanio, A.; Dellière, S.; Fodil, S.; Bretagne, S.; Mégarbane, B. Prevalence of putative invasive pulmonary aspergillosis in critically ill patients with COVID-19. *Lancet Respir. Med.* **2020**, *8*, e48–e49. [CrossRef]
34. Verweij, P.E.; Rijnders, B.J.A.; Brüggemann, R.J.M.; Azoulay, E.; Bassetti, M.; Blot, S.; Calandra, T.; Clancy, C.J.; Cornely, O.A.; Chiller, T.; et al. Review of influenza-associated pulmonary aspergillosis in ICU patients and proposal for a case definition: An expert opinion. *Intensive Care Med.* **2020**, *46*, 1524–1535. [CrossRef]
35. Machado, M.; Estévez, A.; Sánchez-Carrillo, C.; Guinea, J.; Escribano, P.; Alonso, R.; Valerio, M.; Padilla, B.; Bouza, E.; Muñoz, P. Incidence of Candidemia Is Higher in COVID-19 versus Non-COVID-19 Patients, but Not Driven by Intrahospital Transmission. *J. Fungi* **2022**, *8*, 305. [CrossRef]
36. Macauley, P.; Epelbaum, O. Epidemiology and Mycology of Candidaemia in non-oncological medical intensive care unit patients in a tertiary center in the United States: Overall analysis and comparison between non-COVID-19 and COVID-19 cases. *Mycoses* **2021**, *64*, 634–640. [CrossRef]
37. Pappas, P.G.; Kauffman, C.A.; Andes, D.R.; Clancy, C.J.; Marr, K.A.; Ostrosky-Zeichner, L.; Reboli, A.C.; Schuster, M.G.; Vazquez, J.A.; Walsh, T.J.; et al. Clinical Practice Guideline for the Management of Candidiasis: 2016 Update by the Infectious Diseases Society of America. *Clin. Infect. Dis.* **2016**, *62*, e1–e50. [CrossRef] [PubMed]
38. Walton, A.; Muenzer, J.T.; Rasche, D.; Boomer, J.S.; Sato, B.; Brownstein, B.H.; Pachot, A.; Brooks, T.L.; Deych, E.; Shannon, W.D.; et al. Reactivation of Multiple Viruses in Patients with Sepsis. *PLoS ONE* **2014**, *9*, e98819. [CrossRef] [PubMed]
39. Meyer, A.; Buetti, N.; Houhou-Fidouh, N.; Patrier, J.; Abdel-Nabey, M.; Jaquet, P.; Presente, S.; Girard, T.; Sayagh, F.; Ruckly, S.; et al. HSV-1 reactivation is associated with an increased risk of mortality and pneumonia in critically ill COVID-19 patients. *Crit. Care* **2021**, *25*, 1–10. [CrossRef]
40. Saade, A.; Moratelli, G.; Azoulay, E.; Darmon, M. Herpesvirus reactivation during severe COVID-19 and high rate of immune defect. *Infect. Dis. Now* **2021**, *51*, 676–679. [CrossRef]
41. Fuest, K.E.; Erber, J.; Berg-Johnson, W.; Heim, M.; Hoffmann, D.; Kapfer, B.; Kriescher, S.; Ulm, B.; Schmid, R.M.; Rasch, S.; et al. Risk factors for Herpes simplex virus and Cytomegalovirus infections in critically-ill COVID-19 patients. *Multidiscip. Respir. Med.* **2022**, *17*, 815. [CrossRef] [PubMed]
42. Simonnet, A.; Engelmann, I.; Moreau, A.-S.; Garcia, B.; Six, S.; El Kalioubie, A.; Robriquet, L.; Hober, D.; Jourdain, M. High incidence of Epstein–Barr virus, cytomegalovirus, and human-herpes virus-6 reactivations in critically ill patients with COVID-19. *Infect. Dis. Now* **2021**, *51*, 296–299. [CrossRef]
43. Katz, J.; Yue, S.; Xue, W. Herpes simplex and herpes zoster viruses in COVID-19 patients. *Ir. J. Med Sci.* **2021**, *191*, 1093–1097. [CrossRef] [PubMed]

44. Hagel, S.; Scherag, A.; Schuierer, L.; Hoffmann, R.; Luyt, C.-E.; Pletz, M.W.; Kesselmeier, M.; Weis, S. Effect of antiviral therapy on the outcomes of mechanically ventilated patients with herpes simplex virus detected in the respiratory tract: A systematic review and meta-analysis. *Crit. Care* **2020**, *24*, 1–10. [CrossRef] [PubMed]
45. Luyt, C.-E.; Combes, A.; Deback, C.; Aubriot-Lorton, M.-H.; Nieszkowska, A.; Trouillet, J.-L.; Capron, F.; Agut, H.; Gibert, C.; Chastre, J. Herpes Simplex Virus Lung Infection in Patients Undergoing Prolonged Mechanical Ventilation. *Am. J. Respir. Crit. Care Med.* **2007**, *175*, 935–942. [CrossRef] [PubMed]

Journal of
Clinical Medicine

MDPI

Article

Incidence, Outcomes and Risk Factors of Recurrent Ventilator Associated Pneumonia in COVID-19 Patients: A Retrospective Multicenter Study

Ines Gragueb-Chatti [1,*], Hervé Hyvernat [2], Marc Leone [3], Geoffray Agard [1], Noémie Peres [4], Christophe Guervilly [1,5], Mohamed Boucekine [5], Dany Hamidi [2], Laurent Papazian [1,5], Jean Dellamonica [2], Alexandre Lopez [3] and Sami Hraiech [1,5]

1 Service de Médecine Intensive-Réanimation, AP-HM, Hôpital Nord, 13015 Marseille, France
2 Service de Médecine Intensive-Réanimation, CHU Nice, 06202 Nice, France
3 Service d'Anesthésie et de Réanimation, Assistance Publique Hôpitaux de Marseille, Aix Marseille Université, 13015 Marseille, France
4 Service de Réanimation Polyvalente, Centre Hospitalier Intercommunal Toulon—La Seyne sur Mer, 83056 Toulon, France
5 Health Service Research and Quality of Life Center (CEReSS), Aix-Marseille Université, 27 Boulevard Jean-Moulin, 13005 Marseille, France
* Correspondence: ines.gragueb-chatti@ap-hm.fr; Tel.: +33-4-91-96-58-36; Fax: +33-4-91-96-58-37

Abstract: Background: High incidence of ventilator associated pneumonia (VAP) has been reported in critically ill patients with COVID-19. Among these patients, we aimed to assess the incidence, outcomes and risk factors of VAP recurrences. Methods: We conducted an observational retrospective study in three French intensive care units (ICUs). Patients admitted for a documented COVID-19 from March 2020 to May 2021 and requiring mechanical ventilation (MV) for ≥48 h were included. The study main outcome was the incidence of VAP recurrences. Secondary outcomes were the duration of MV, ICU and hospital length of stay and mortality according to VAP and recurrences. We also assessed the factors associated with VAP recurrences. Results: During the study period, 398 patients met the inclusion criteria. A total of 236 (59%) of them had at least one VAP episode during their ICU stay and 109 (46%) of these patients developed at least one recurrence. The incidence of VAP recurrence considering death and extubation as competing events was 29.6% (IC = [0.250–0.343]). Seventy-eight percent of recurrences were due to the same bacteria (relapses). Patients with a VAP recurrence had a longer duration of MV as compared with one VAP and no VAP patients (41 (25–56) vs. 16 (8–30) and 10 (5–18) days; $p < 0.001$) and a longer ICU length of stay (46 (29–66) vs. 22 (12–36) and 14 (9–25) days; $p < 0.001$). The 90-day mortality was higher in the recurrence group as compared with the no VAP group only (31.2 vs. 21.0% ($p = 0.021$)). In a multivariate analysis including bacterial co-infection at admission, the use of immunosuppressive therapies and the bacteria responsible for the first VAP episode, the duration of MV was the only factor independently associated with VAP recurrence. Conclusion: In COVID-19 associated respiratory failure, recurrences affected 46% of patients with a first episode of VAP. VAP recurrences were mainly relapses and were associated with a prolonged duration of MV and ICU length of stay but not with a higher mortality. MV duration was the only factor associated with recurrences.

Keywords: COVID-19; ICU; ventilator-associated pneumonia; acute respiratory distress syndrome; recurrence of VAP

Citation: Gragueb-Chatti, I.; Hyvernat, H.; Leone, M.; Agard, G.; Peres, N.; Guervilly, C.; Boucekine, M.; Hamidi, D.; Papazian, L.; Dellamonica, J.; et al. Incidence, Outcomes and Risk Factors of Recurrent Ventilator Associated Pneumonia in COVID-19 Patients: A Retrospective Multicenter Study. *J. Clin. Med.* **2022**, *11*, 7097. https://doi.org/10.3390/jcm11237097

Academic Editor: Ulrich Hermann Frey

Received: 10 October 2022
Accepted: 25 November 2022
Published: 30 November 2022

1. Background

Patients admitted to the intensive care unit (ICU) because of severe forms of Coronavirus Disease 2019 (COVID-19) require invasive mechanical ventilation (MV) in up to 80% of cases [1]. Unexpectedly high rates of ventilator associated pneumonia (VAP) have been reported among these patients, reaching 50 to 80% according to the series [2,3]. Specific features of SARS-CoV-2 pneumonia seem to be involved as COVID-19 patients develop more VAP than do Influenza patients, regardless the duration of MV [3]. Several mechanisms have been suggested to explain this increase in nosocomial bacterial pneumonia, mainly the immune system impairment due to SARS-CoV-2 infection [4,5], the use of corticosteroids [5–7], and the high incidence of ARDS with prolonged MV and recourse to prone positioning [8,9].

Some series also pointed out the recurrence of several episodes of VAP in the same patients [10,11]. Recurrence was most often due to the same pathogen (relapse), despite a well conducted antibiotic treatment [10] and was associated with a poor prognosis. However, these data were limited to patients under veno-veinous extracorporeal membrane oxygenation (ECMO). No study specifically addressed the question of VAP recurrences in patients with severe SARS-CoV-2 pneumonia despite the use of broad spectrum and prolonged antibiotic treatments they are associated with [10–12].

We aimed to describe clinical and microbial characteristics of patients with a VAP recurrence during COVID-19. Primary outcome was to determine the incidence of VAP recurrences. Secondary outcomes were to describe their microbiological features, evaluate their impact on the duration of MV, ICU and hospital length of stay and mortality and to bring to light potential risk factors exposing to VAP recurrence.

2. Methods

2.1. Study Design and Population

We conducted an observational retrospective study in three ICUs from two university hospitals in Southern France. From 1 March 2020 to 1 May 2021, all patients aged 18 or older, admitted for acute respiratory failure related to a documented SARS-CoV-2 pneumonia (from a nasopharyngeal or pulmonary sample RT-PCR) and requiring invasive MV for at least 48 h were included. Patients for whom withholding of treatments was decided during the first 48 h after ICU admission, aged under 18, deprived of liberty or without social protection, refusing (patients or relatives) the use of medical data collected for routine care were not included.

2.2. Definitions

VAP Diagnosis

VAP was diagnosed in patients having received MV for at least 48 h when the following criteria were met [13,14]:

- New or progressive persistent infiltration on chest radiograph;
- At least two of the following: new onset of fever, purulent endotracheal aspirate, leukocytosis or leucopenia, increased minute ventilation, arterial oxygenation decline, need for increased vasopressor infusion to maintain blood pressure (for patients with ARDS, for whom demonstration of radiologic deterioration is difficult, at least two of the preceding criteria sufficed);
- A positive quantitative or qualitative culture from broncho-alveolar lavage (BAL), protected distal sample (PDS) or endotracheal aspirate (ETA).

A positive bacterial culture on a respiratory sample without clinical sign of pneumonia and without antibiotic treatment initiated was considered as a colonization.

2.3. Bacterial Co-Infection at ICU Admission

A bacterial co-infection was diagnosed when an invasive (BAL, PDS, ETA, blood cultures) or non-invasive (sputum sample, multiplex PCR, *Streptococcus pneumoniae* or *Legionnella pneumophila* antigenuria) sample was positive before ICU admission or within the 48 h following it.

2.4. Relapse and Recurrence of VAP

Recurrence of VAP was defined as a new onset following a regression of clinical signs (fever, expectorations, and vasopressor infusion), inflammatory biomarkers and infiltration on chest radiography after a complete adequate antibiotic treatment (at least one antibiotic active against the documented bacteria). VAP recurrence was diagnosed on clinical signs reappearance and at least one bacterial species growth at a significant concentration from respiratory samples. Relapse was defined as a recurrence involving at least one of the initial causative bacteria; otherwise, it was considered a superinfection.

2.5. Baseline Assessment and Data Collection

Data were collected from the patients' electronic medical file. Demographic characteristics, comorbidities, severity at ICU admission, date of SARS-CoV-2 RT-PCR positivity, date of ICU admission, date of intubation and invasive MV, need for ECMO, antiviral treatment, initial bacterial co-infection and antibiotics received at ICU admission, VAP with microbiological documentation and recurrences, antibiotics received during the ICU stay, duration of antibiotics treatment, duration of total invasive MV, ICU and hospital stay, status at day 28 (from the start of ICU hospitalization), day 90 (includes after hospital discharge), ICU and hospital mortality were obtained. The use of immunomodulatory/immunosuppressive (IS) therapies was also recorded:

Dexamethasone (at 6 or 12 mg per day) [15]
Methylprednisolone for persistent ARDS as described elsewhere [16]
Hydrocortisone (at 200 mg per day)
Interleukine-6 (Il-6) receptor antagonist (Tocilizumab) [17]
Interleukin-1(Il-1) receptor antagonist (Anakinra) [18]
Janus Kinases (JAK) receptor antagonist (Ruxolitinib) [18]
The combination of several of them during the same ICU stay

2.6. Antibiotic Treatment

Empiric antibiotic therapy was started in case of VAP suspicion according to national and international recommendations [19–22]. De-escalation was performed if possible as soon as the results of microbiological investigations performed were available [21,23].

2.7. Management of Antibiotic Treatment

Antibiotic administration through prolonged infusions was used as it was part of the routine care in each of the three ICUs. Empirical antibiotic treatment was considered adequate when the patient received at least one antibiotic active against the responsible pathogen [23].

Therapeutic drug monitoring was performed according to physicians' decision.

2.8. Study Outcomes

The primary outcome was the incidence of VAP recurrences. The secondary outcomes were the microbiological description of VAP recurrences, the percentage of antibiotic target attainment (serum concentration above 4 times the minimal inhibitory concentration (MIC) of documented bacteria), the evolution towards lung abscess, the impact of VAP and recurrences on the duration of invasive MV, ICU and hospital length of stay and mortality and the factors associated with VAP recurrences.

2.9. Statistical Analysis

Statistical analysis was performed using SPSS Version 20 (IBM SPSS Inc., Chicago, IL, USA).

Continuous variables are expressed as mean ± standard deviation (SD) or as median with interquartile range, and categorical variables are reported as count and percentages. Comparisons between groups were performed using Student's *t*-test or Mann–Whitney U as appropriate. Comparisons of percentages were performed using Chi-square test or (Fisher's exact test, as appropriate).

We performed a multivariate logistic regression analysis including non collinear variables with $p < 0.2$ in univariate analysis to determine the influence of clinical parameters on VAP recurrence.

Fine–Gray model was used to estimate the cumulative incidence of VAP recurrence considering death and extubation as competing risks [24]. Analysis was performed using the cuminc function from cmprsk r package.

We confirmed impact of variables on timing of VAP incidence by a COX model and constructed Kaplan–Meier curves. Curves were compared with the Log Rank test.

The statistical significance was defined as $p < 0.05$.

3. Results

3.1. Patients' Characteristics at ICU Admission

Study flow chart is presented in Figure 1. A total of 398 patients were included in the final analysis. Table 1 shows the repartition of patients according to the occurrence of VAP. During the ICU stay, 162 (40.7%) patients did not develop VAP (no VAP group), 127 (31.9%) had a single VAP episode (1 VAP group) and 109 (27.4%) had a recurrence of VAP (2 or more episodes, recurrence group). A total of 236 (59%) patients had at least one VAP and 109 (46%) of these patients developed at least one recurrence (65 patients had 2 VAP and 44 patients had 3 VAP). The recurrence was diagnosed using BAL and ETA in 44 and 65 cases, respectively. In the recurrence group, the median delay from first to second VAP was 11.7 [5.0–17.0] days. Admissions were spread during the first three waves of pandemics in France. A total of 264 (66.3%) patients received empirical antibiotics at ICU admission without any difference between groups. An initial co-infection was documented in only 44 (11.1%) patients and was more frequent in patients that presented a VAP recurrence than in one VAP or no VAP groups (17.4% vs. 10.2% and 7.4% respectively; $p = 0.035$). In the recurrence group, V/V ECMO was more frequently used than in the one VAP and no VAP patients (34.9% vs. 14.2% and 13.6%; $p < 0.001$).

ECMO: extracorporeal membrane oxygenation; ICU: intensive care unit; IQR: interquartile range; IMV: invasive mechanical ventilation; SAPS II: simplified acute physiologic Score II; SD: standard deviation; SOFA: sequential organ failure assessment; VAP: ventilator-associated pneumonia.

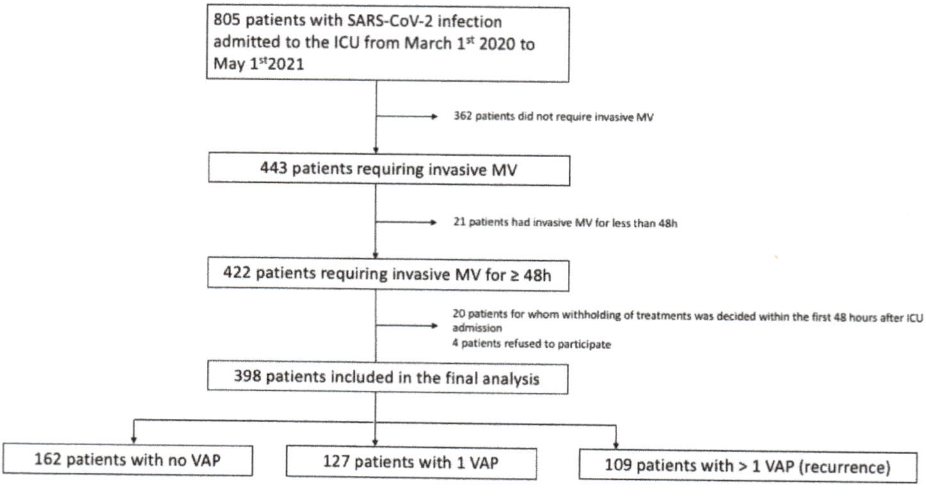

Figure 1. Study flow chart. ICU: intensive care unit; MV: mechanical ventilation; VAP: ventilator-associated pneumonia.

Table 1. Patients' main characteristics at ICU admission according to the occurrence of VAP.

	TOTAL (n = 398)	0 VAP (n = 162)	1 VAP (n = 127)	>1 VAP (n = 109)	p
Age, years ± SD	65 ± 12	63 ± 12	66 ± 12	66 ± 10	0.445
Male, n (%)	287 (72.1)	112 (69.1)	93 (73.2)	82 (75.2)	0.517
SAPS II, mean ± SD	40 (31–51)	40 (31–45)	40 (33–48)	42(34–51)	0.369
SOFA, mean ± SD	5 (3–8)	5 (3–7)	5 (3–8)	6 (4–8)	0.479
COMORBIDITIES, n (%)					
Chronic Heart Failure	71 (17.8)	28 (17.3)	27 (21.3)	16 (14.7)	0.408
Chronic respiratory failure	48 (12.1)	20 (12.3)	16 (12.6)	12 (11)	0.923
Chronic kidney failure	29 (7.3)	9 (5.6)	12 (9.4)	8 (7.3)	0.450
Hypertension	193 (48.5)	80 (49.4)	58 (45.7)	55 (50.5)	0.731
Diabetes mellitus	140 (35.2)	51 (31.5)	45 (35.4)	44 (40.4)	0.323
Smoker	93 (23.4)	45 (27.8)	22 (17.3)	26 (23.9)	0.114
Obesity	161 (40.5)	72 (44.4)	43 (33.9)	46 (42.2)	0.174
History of neoplasm	42 (10.6)	15 (9.3)	15 (11.8)	12 (11)	0.766
Immunosuppression	39 (9.8)	15 (9.3)	11 (8.7)	13 (11.9)	0.671
Admission periods, n (%)					
First wave	67 (16.8)	27 (16.7)	23 (18.1)	17 (15.6)	0.874
Second wave	144 (36.1)	53 (32.7)	48 (37.8)	43 (39.4)	0.474
Third wave	187 (47.0)	82 (50.6)	56 (44.0)	49 (45.0)	0.480
Time from hospital to ICU admission, days, median (IQR)	3 (0–3)	3.2 (0–4)	1.7 (0–2)	2.9 (0–3)	0.68
IMV, n (%)	76 (19.1)	29 (17.9)	27 (21.3)	20 (18.3)	0.93
ECMO, n (%)	78 (19.6)	22 (13.6)	18 (14.2)	38 (34.9)	**<0.001**
Antiviral agent [a], n (%)	134 (33.7)	43 (26.5)	46 (36.2)	45 (41.3)	**0.032**
Antibiotic treatment, n (%)	264 (66.3)	114 (70.4)	80 (63)	70 (64.2)	0.21
Documented co-infection, n (%)	44 (11.1)	12 (7.4)	13 (10.2)	19 (17.4)	**0.035**

Data are presented as median and interquartile range or absolute value and percentage. p values in bold were considered statistically significant. [a] remdesivir, lopinavir or ritonavir.

3.2. VAP and Recurrence Incidence

Figure 2 shows the cumulative incidence of VAP recurrence, considering death and duration of MV (extubation) as competing events. The incidence of VAP recurrence was 29.6% (IC = [0.250–0.343]).

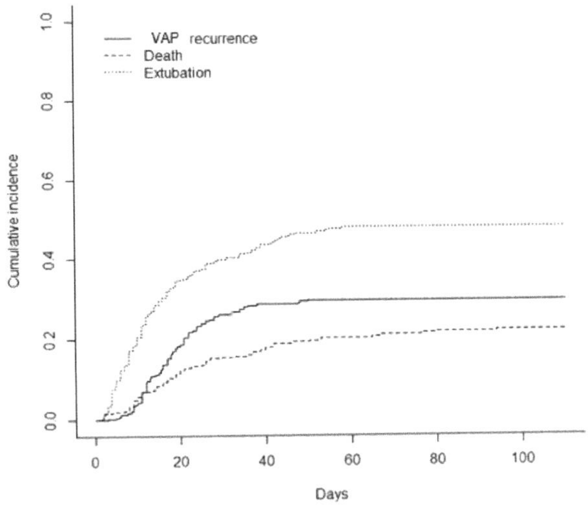

Figure 2. Estimated cumulative incidence of ventilator-associated pneumonia (VAP) recurrence considering death and extubation as competing events. VAP: ventilator-associated pneumonia.

3.3. Use of Immunosuppressive Therapies during the ICU Stays

Table 2 shows the use of IS therapies in each group. Patients in the recurrence group were more often treated with methylprednisolone for persistent ARDS and received more frequently a combination of two IS as compared with 1 VAP group and no VAP group ($p < 0.01$).

Table 2. Immunomodulator/immunosuppressive (IS) therapies received during the ICU stay.

	TOTAL (n = 398)	0 VAP (n = 162)	1 VAP (n = 127)	>1 VAP (n = 109)
IS therapy, n (%)	338 (84.9)	129 (79.6) [a]	**108 (85)**	**101 (92.7)** [b]
Dexamethasone, n (%)	324 (81.4)	129 (79.6)	103 (81.1)	92 (84.4)
Methylprednisolone, n (%)	104 (26.1)	25 (15.4) [a]	**26 (20.5)** [a]	**53 (48.6)** [b,c]
IL-1 receptor antagonist, n (%)	15 (3.8)	4 (2.5)	4 (3.1)	7 (6.4)
JAK receptor antagonist, n (%)	19 (4.8)	4 (2.5)	8 (6.3)	7 (6.4)
IL-6 receptor antagonist, n (%) [c]	75 (18.8)	**12 (7.4)** [a,c]	**31 (24.4)** [b]	32 (29.4) [b]
Combination of 2 IS, n (%) [d]	193 (48.5)	**51 (31.5)** [a,c]	**63 (49.6)** [a,b]	**79 (72.5)** [b,c]

Values in bold were considered statistically significant. Data are presented as absolute value and percentage. ICU: intensive care unit; IL-1: interleukine 1; IL-6: interleukine 6; IS: immunosuppressive; JAK: janus kinase; VAP: ventilator-associated pneumonia. [a] $p < 0.01$ vs. >1 VAP. [b] $p < 0.01$ vs. 0 VAP. [c] $p < 0.01$ vs. 1 VAP.

3.4. Microbiological and Pharmacological Results

Table 3 depicts the micro-organisms responsible of VAP. Gram-negative bacteria (55.9%), especially *Enterobacteriaceae*, were predominant during the first VAP episode. Non-fermenting Gram-negative bacteria (*Pseudomonas aeruginosa* and *Stenotrophomonas maltophilia*) were majority during recurrences (54.2% of gram-negative bacilli). Gram-positive pathogens (25.7%) were mainly methicillin-susceptible *Staphylococcus aureus* (MSSA) and *Enterococcus* spp.

Table 3. Micro-organisms responsible for VAP (1st episode and recurrences).

	1st VAP (n = 338)	2nd VAP (n = 165)	3rd VAP (n = 69)
Gram-negative bacilli, n (%)	189 (55.9)	101 (61.2)	48 (69.6)
Enterobacteriaceae	139	60	22
Non-fermenting GNB	50	41	26
Gram-positive cocci, n (%)	87 (25.7)	31 (18.8)	8 (11.6)
MSSA	50	21	5
MRSA	6	3	1
Enterococcus spp.	14	6	2
Streptococcus spp.	17	1	0
Polymicrobial, n (%)	62 (18.3)	33 (20.0)	13 (18.9)
Antibiotic-multiresistant bacteria, n	11 (3.2)	14 (8.5)	14 (20.0)
ESBLE-producing Enterobacteriaceae	8	11	10
Carbapenem-resistant *enterobacteriaceae*	1	2	1
Multi-drug resistant *Pseudomonas*	2	1	3

n refers to the number of VAP episodes. Data are presented as absolute value and percentage of micro-organisms. ESBLE: extended spectrum beta-lactamase; GNB: gram negative bacilli; MRSA methicillin-resistant Staphylococcus aureus, MSSA methicillin-sensitive Staphylococcus aureus; VAP: ventilator-associated pneumonia

Seventy-eight percent of recurrences were relapses—i.e., involved the same bacteria—despite appropriate treatment of the preceding VAP.

Therapeutic drug monitoring was performed in 69 (54%) of 127 patients during first VAP episode. Serum antibiotic concentrations reached therapeutic range according to MIC90 in 50 (72.5%) patients. Noteworthy, the patients with VAP recurrence developed more frequently lung abscesses, as compared with those with one VAP episode (16 (14.7%) vs. 8 (6.2%); $p < 0.001$).

Multi-drug resistant is defined as non-susceptibility to ≥1 drug in ≥3 antimicrobial categories.

3.5. Clinical Outcomes

Table 4 shows the clinical outcomes of patients according to the occurrence of VAP and recurrence. A total of 19 patients were lost to follow-up. The recurrence group had increased duration of invasive MV (41 (25–56) vs. 16 (8–30) and 10 (5–18) days; $p < 0.001$) and ICU stay duration as compared with one VAP and no VAP groups (46 (29–66) vs. 22 (12–36) and 14 (9–25) days; $p < 0.001$). The 90-day mortality was higher in the recurrence group as compared with the no VAP group, 31.2 vs. 21.0% ($p = 0.021$). There was no mortality difference between the recurrence group and the 1 VAP group ($p = 0.41$).

Table 4. Clinical outcomes according to the occurrence of VAP and recurrence.

	TOTAL ($n = 398$)	**0 VAP** ($n = 162$)	**1 VAP** ($n = 127$)	**>1 VAP** ($n = 109$)	p
OUTCOMES, days, median (IQR)					
Duration of mechanical ventilation	17 (8–36)	10 (5–18)	16 (8–30)	41 (25–56)	**<0.001**
VFD at D28	9 (0–19)	17 (8–22)	11 (0–19)	0 (0–1)	**<0.001**
VFD at D60	41 (21–51)	48 (40–54)	42.5 (28–51)	17 (0–33)	**<0.001**
ICU length of stay	23 (12–42)	14 (9–25)	22 (12–36)	46 (29–66)	**<0.001**
Hospital length of stay	29 (18–49)	22 (14–36)	29 (17–44)	53 (32–75)	**<0.001**
MORTALITY OUTCOMES, n (%)					
ICU mortality	111 (27.9)	32 (19.8)	43 (33.9)	36 (33.0)	**0.011**
D28 mortality	69 (17.3)	30 (18.5)	30 (23.6)	9 (8.3)	**0.006**
D90 mortality	114 (28.6)	34 (21.0)	46 (36.2)	34 (31.2)	**0.021**

p values in bold were considered statistically significant. Data are presented as median and interquartile range or absolute value and percentage ICU: intensive care unit; IQR: interquartile range; VAP: ventilator-associated pneumonia; VFD: ventilator free days.

The predicted probability of death at day 90 was 33.9% (IC [26%; 44.2%]) for a patient with no VAP, 33.5% (IC [25.6%; 43.9%]) with one VAP episode and 47.8% (IC [21.9%; 100%]) for a patient with a VAP recurrence.

3.6. Factors Associated with VAP Recurrences

Factors associated with VAP recurrence were evaluated among patients with at least one VAP episode (one VAP and recurrence groups, $n = 236$). Age, SAPS2 score, SOFA score at ICU admission, obesity, bacterial co-infection at ICU admission, IS therapy, antibiotic target attainment, type of bacteria responsible for the first VAP, and duration of invasive MV prior the first VAP were included in the univariate analysis. Variables that reached p values of less than 0.20 in univariate analysis were included in the multivariate analysis (Table 5).

The duration of MV was the only variable independently associated with VAP recurrence. The specific role of IS therapies on the timing of second VAP occurrence was assessed using a Cox regression model. We used univariate Cox model testing: (a) all IS therapies, (b) only steroidal IS or (c) only non-steroidal IS on delay of VAP relapse. The use of steroidal IS (i.e., dexamethasone or hydrocortisone or methylprednisolone) delayed the second VAP by a mean of 5 days (20.0 [17.7–22.2] vs. 14.7 [12.6–16.7] days; $p = 0.002$) (Figure 3a). Non-steroidal IS treatment shortened the delay of second VAP occurrence by a mean of 5 days (15.1 [12.6–17.7] vs. 20.0 [17.8–22.2] days; $p = 0.006$) (Figure 3b).

Table 5. Factors associated with VAP recurrence in univariate and multivariate analysis.

	Univariate Analysis			Multivariate Analysis		
	1 VAP (n = 127)	**Recurrence (n = 109)**	p	**Odds Ratio**	**95% CI**	p
		Variable				
Age, y	63 ± 12	64 ± 10	0.54			
SAPS 2	40 (33–48)	42 (34–51)	0.13	1	0.98–1.03	0.62
SOFA [a]	5 (3–8)	6 (4–8)	0.20			
Obesity, n (%)	43 (34)	46 (42)	0.22			
IS treatment (at least one), n (%)	106 (83)	101 (93)	0.06	0.5	0.18–1.39	0.19
Steroidal IS, n (%)	42 (33)	74 (68)	<0.001	0.75	0.37–1.52	0.43
Non steroidal IS, n (%)	39 (31)	39 (36)	0.46			
Association of 2 IS, n (%)	62 (49)	79 (73)	<0.001	0.66	0.34–1.27	0.21
Bacterial co-infection at ICU admission, n (%)	12 (9)	19 (17)	0.08	0.64	0.26–1.56	0.32
Antibiotic target attainment [b]	20 (69)	30 (75)	0.07	0.94	0.43–2.09	0.89
Duration of MV	16 (8–30)	41 (25–56)	<0.001	1.06	1.04–1.08	**<0.001**
		First VAP documentation				
Gram positive Cocci	51	42	0.72			
Enterobacteriaceae	60	61	0.22			
Non-fermenting negative Gram Bacilli	24	23	0.72			

p values in bold were considered statistically significant. Quantitative variable are presented as mean ± standard deviation or median and interquartile range. [a] On the day of ICU admission. [b] n = 29 for 1 VAP group and n = 40 for recurrence group. CI: confidence interval; ICU: intensive care unit; IS: immunosuppressive/immunomodulatory; MV: mechanical ventilation; SAPS2: Simplified Acute Physiology Score 2.

Concerning the produced product of the time (delay of VAP relapse) by the covariable, p value was, respectively, 0.276 for all IS, 0.923 for steroidal IS and 0.220 for non-steroidal IS, indicating for all models no gross violation of proportional hazard of Cox model.

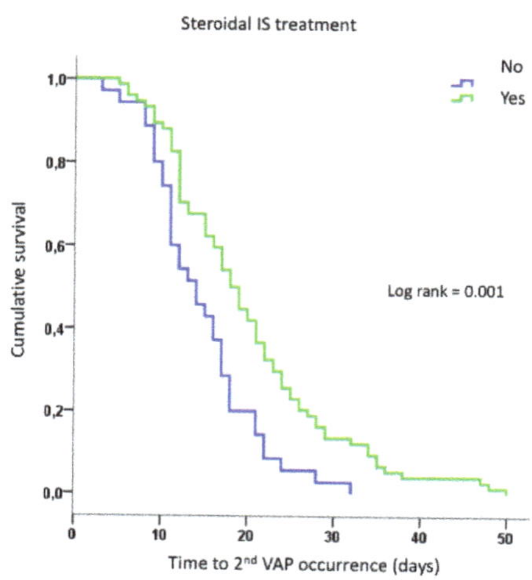

(a)

Figure 3. *Cont.*

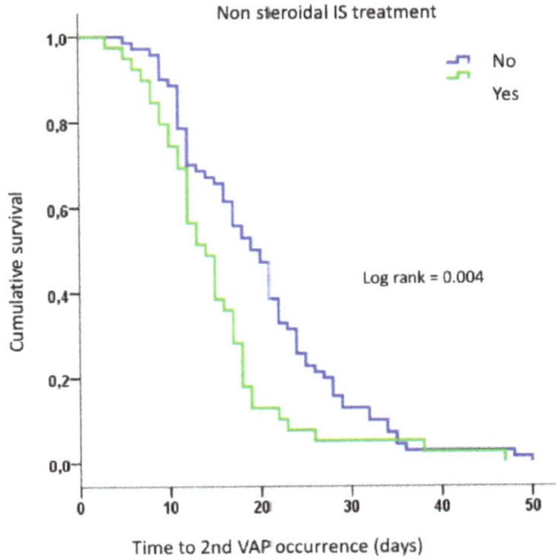

(**b**)

Figure 3. (**a**): Cumulated survival probability before 2nd VAP occurrence according to the use of steroidal IS treatment (subjects were censored at the time of VAP recurrence). (**b**): Cumulated survival probability before 2nd VAP occurrence according to the use of non-steroidal IS treatment (subjects were censored at the time of VAP recurrence). IS: immunosuppressive; VAP: ventilator-associated pneumonia.

4. Discussion

In this cohort specifically addressing the question of VAP recurrences during COVID-19 pneumonia, more than half of the patients developed at least one VAP episode and 46% of these patients had at least one recurrence. The incidence of VAP recurrence considering death and extubation as competing events was 29.6%. *Enterobacteriaceae* and non-fermenting Gram-negative bacteria were mainly involved and 78% of VAP recurrences were relapses. Recurrences were associated with longer duration of MV and ICU length of stay, although 90-day mortality was not affected. The duration of MV was the only factor independently associated with recurrences, even after considering the use of immunosuppressive therapies.

The high rate of VAP described in our series is in line with a recent review showing that in COVID-19 patients, VAP incidence ranged from 21 to 85% [12]. In a large European cohort, Rouzé et al. [3] reported a 51% incidence, significantly higher than in Influenza patients. As a comparison, a 29% rate of VAP in non-COVID-19 ARDS patients was described [21]. Few data are available on VAP recurrences, with rates ranging from 8 to 25% [3,25–28] in studies not designed to explore specifically this endpoint. In a highly selected population of patients under V/V ECMO, Luyt et al. reported up to 59% of recurrences [10].

We found that prolonged invasive MV was the only factor independently associated with the risk of VAP recurrence. Although it is difficult to characterize the causal relationship between VAP and MV duration, several studies showed that COVID-19 patients have an increased risk of VAP, independently of the duration of MV [3,10,28]. We assessed here the role of immunosuppressive treatments. Previous studies suggested that dexamethasone alone was not associated with an increased risk of VAP [2]. In our cohort, the association of two IS therapies was used in 48.5% of patients, mainly a combination of dexamethasone and tocilizumab and/or methylprednisolone for persistent ARDS. However, neither the treatment with one nor the combination of several IS were independently associated with an increased VAP recurrence risk. This is of particular interest considering that dexamethasone was a part of standard of care and tocilizumab was largely used in

ICU patients [6,15,17,29]. Noteworthy, the use of non-steroidal IS therapies was associated with an earlier development of VAP recurrence. IL-6 antagonists cause a transient but long-lasting immunosuppressive state, which may favor the occurrence of bacterial superinfections, such as VAP. Conversely, the use of steroids was associated with a delayed recurrence of VAP.

As described in the series from Luyt et al. [10], we found that 78% of recurrences were relapses, mainly involving *Enterobacteriaceae*. This result questions the efficacy of first VAP antibiotic treatment. However, when therapeutic drug monitoring was performed, target attainment was reached in 72.5% of patients. It has been suggested that pulmonary vascular endothelial inflammation and subsequent thrombosis might make the lung parenchyma a favorable substrate for bacterial growth and prevent antimicrobial penetration [30,31]. Altogether, our findings highlight the need for secondary infection monitoring, [25–27]. The high rate of relapses in our patients also questions about the best duration of antibiotic treatment in COVID-19 patients with bacterial co-infection. This seems a critical issue since we observed an unexpected high number of lung abscesses (14.7%) in the recurrence group, also reported in a previous cohort [32]. In our series, all patients with a first VAP were treated for 7 consecutive days, as recommended [33–36]. The so-called COVID-19 related "immunoparalysis" [37] could also explain the high rate of relapses. Decreased mHLA-DR expression is associated with the development of severe respiratory failure, and presumably may contribute to pronounced susceptibility to bacterial superinfections [34].

VAP recurrence was associated with a prolonged invasive MV duration and ICU length of stay although it did not affect 90-day mortality. Previous studies have shown that VAP during COVID-19 ARDS were associated with a higher mortality [38,39]. As it has been proposed in non-COVID-19 patients, VAP seems associated with prolonged duration of invasive MV and prolonged ICU stay, whereas mortality is mainly driven by patients' underlying conditions and illness severity [8].

Our study has several limitations. First, the retrospective design with inherently associated bias. Second, the low rate of patients with serum antibiotic concentration monitoring prevents determining the effect of under-dosing in relapses. Finally, the strong association between patient's severity, duration of MV and the use of immunosuppressive treatments hardens to strongly conclude about VAP recurrence risk factors. In our analysis, the weight of invasive MV duration over-rode other variables. In particular, the role of immunosuppressive therapies deserves to be more deeply explored.

5. Conclusions

In this series, we found that nearly half of patients under invasive MV for COVID-19 pneumonia with a first VAP episode developed recurrences, which were relapses in most cases. Patients with a VAP recurrence had a longer duration of invasive MV and ICU length of stay but not a higher mortality. MV duration was the only factor associated with VAP recurrences.

Author Contributions: S.H., I.G.-C., H.H., G.A., N.P., A.L. and D.H. collected and analyzed the data. S.H., I.G.-C., C.G., L.P., M.L. and J.D. analyzed and interpreted more precisely the data. M.B., C.G. and S.H. performed the statistical analysis. S.H., I.G.-C. and L.P. wrote the manuscript. All authors have read and agreed to the published version of the manuscript.

Funding: The authors received no funding for this work.

Institutional Review Board Statement: The study was approved by the French Intensive Care Society (SRLF) Ethics Committee (Commission d'Ethique de la SRLF, reference CE SRLF 21-06) which waived the need for written consent according to French legislation. The study was also declared and approved by the "Portail d'Accès aux Données de Santé, Assistance Publique-Hôpitaux de Marseille" (Registration number PADS20-366).

Informed Consent Statement: Patients and their relatives were informed of the possibility to use their medical data for retrospective studies and their opposition was researched. The study was approved by the French Intensive Care Society (SRLF) Ethics Committee (Commission d'Ethique de la SRLF, reference CE SRLF 21-06) which waived the need for written consent according to French legislation. The study was also declared and approved by the "Portail d'Accès aux Données de Santé, Assistance Publique-Hôpitaux de Marseille" (Registration number PADS20-366).

Data Availability Statement: The datasets used and/or analyzed during the current study are available from the corresponding author on reasonable request.

Conflicts of Interest: The authors declare no conflict of interest.

List of Abbreviations

ARDS	acute respiratory distress syndrome
BAL	broncho-alveolar lavage
ECMO	extracorporeal membrane oxygenation
ETA	endotracheal aspirate
IL-1	interleukine 1
IL-6	interleukine 6
ICU	intensive care unit
IS	immunosuppressive
JAK	janus kinase
MSSA	methicillin-susceptible *Staphylococcus aureus*
MV	mechanical ventilation
PSD	protected distal sample
PCR	polymerase chain reaction
RT-PCR	reverse transcription polymerase chain reaction
SAPS II	simplified acute physiologic Score II
SOFA	sequential organ failure assessment
SRLF	société de réanimation de langue française
VAP	ventilator-associated pneumonia
VFD	ventilator free days

References

1. COVID-ICU Group on behalf of the REVA Network and the COVID-ICU Investigators. Clinical characteristics and day-90 outcomes of 4244 critically ill adults with COVID-19: A prospective cohort study. *Intensive Care Med.* **2021**, *47*, 60–73. [CrossRef] [PubMed]
2. Gragueb-Chatti, I.; Lopez, A.; Hamidi, D.; Guervilly, C.; Loundou, A.; Daviet, F.; Cassir, N.; Papazian, L.; Forel, J.-M.; Leone, M.; et al. Impact of dexamethasone on the incidence of ventilator-associated pneumonia and blood stream infections in COVID-19 patients requiring invasive mechanical ventilation: A multicenter retrospective study. *Ann. Intensive Care* **2021**, *11*, 87. [CrossRef] [PubMed]
3. Rouzé, A.; Martin-Loeches, I.; Povoa, P.; Makris, D.; Artigas, A.; Bouchereau, M.; Lambiotte, F.; Metzelard, M.; Cuchet, P.; Geronimi, C.B.; et al. Relationship between SARS-CoV-2 infection and the incidence of ventilator-associated lower respiratory tract infections: A European multicenter cohort study. *Intensive Care Med.* **2021**, *47*, 188–198. [CrossRef] [PubMed]
4. Hall, M.W.; Joshi, I.; Leal, L.; Ooi, E.E. Immune Immunomodulation in Coronavirus Disease 2019 (COVID-19): Strategic Considerations for Personalized Therapeutic Intervention. *Clin. Infect. Dis.* **2022**, *74*, 144–148. [CrossRef]
5. Cour, M.; Simon, M.; Argaud, L.; Monneret, G.; Venet, F. Effects of dexamethasone on immune dysfunction and ventilator-associated pneumonia in COVID-19 acute respiratory distress syndrome: An observational study. *J. Intensive Care* **2021**, *9*, 64. [CrossRef]
6. The WHO Rapid Evidence Appraisal for COVID-19 Therapies (REACT) Working Group. Association between Administration of Systemic Corticosteroids and Mortality among Critically Ill Patients with COVID-19: A Meta-analysis. *JAMA* **2020**, *324*, 1330. [CrossRef]
7. Tomazini, B.M.; Maia, I.S.; Cavalcanti, A.B.; Berwanger, O.; Rosa, R.G.; Veiga, V.C.; Avezum, A.; Lopes, R.D.; Bueno, F.R.; Silva, M.V.A.O.; et al. Effect of Dexamethasone on Days Alive and Ventilator-Free in Patients with Moderate or Severe Acute Respiratory Distress Syndrome and COVID-19: The CoDEX Randomized Clinical Trial. *JAMA* **2020**, *324*, 1307. [CrossRef]
8. Papazian, L.; Klompas, M.; Luyt, C.-E. Ventilator-associated pneumonia in adults: A narrative review. *Intensive Care Med.* **2020**, *46*, 888–906. [CrossRef]

9. Ferrando, C.; Suarez-Sipmann, F.; Mellado-Artigas, R.; Hernández, M.; Gea, A.; Arruti, E.; Aldecoa, C.; Martínez-Pallí, G.; Martínez-González, M.A.; Slutsky, A.S.; et al. Clinical features, ventilatory management, and outcome of ARDS caused by COVID-19 are similar to other causes of ARDS. *Intensive Care Med.* **2020**, *46*, 2200–2211. [CrossRef]
10. Luyt, C.-E.; Sahnoun, T.; Gautier, M.; Vidal, P.; Burrel, S.; Pineton de Chambrun, M.; Chommeloux, J.; Desnos, C.; Arzoine, J.; Nieszkowska, A.; et al. Ventilator-associated pneumonia in patients with SARS-CoV-2-associated acute respiratory distress syndrome requiring ECMO: A retrospective cohort study. *Ann. Intensive Care* **2020**, *10*, 158. [CrossRef]
11. Gregorova, M.; Morse, D.; Brignoli, T.; Steventon, J.; Hamilton, F.; Albur, M.; Arnold, D.; Thomas, M.; Halliday, A.; Baum, H.; et al. Post-acute COVID-19 associated with evidence of bystander T-cell activation and a recurring antibiotic-resistant bacterial pneumonia. *eLife* **2020**, *9*, e63430. [CrossRef]
12. Fumagalli, J.; Panigada, M.; Klompas, M.; Berra, L. Ventilator-associated pneumonia among SARS-CoV-2 acute respiratory distress syndrome patients. *Curr. Opin. Crit. Care* **2022**, *28*, 74–82. [CrossRef]
13. Kalil, A.C.; Metersky, M.L.; Klompas, M.; Muscedere, J.; Sweeney, D.A.; Palmer, L.B.; Napolitano, L.M.; O'Grady, N.P.; Bartlett, J.G.; Carratalà, J.; et al. Management of Adults with Hospital-acquired and Ventilator-associated Pneumonia: 2016 Clinical Practice Guidelines by the Infectious Diseases Society of America and the American Thoracic Society. *Clin. Infect. Dis.* **2016**, *63*, e61–e111. [CrossRef]
14. François, B.; Laterre, P.-F.; Luyt, C.-E.; Chastre, J. The challenge of ventilator-associated pneumonia diagnosis in COVID-19 patients. *Crit. Care* **2020**, *24*, 289. [CrossRef]
15. The RECOVERY Collaborative Group. Dexamethasone in Hospitalized Patients with COVID-19. *N. Engl. J. Med.* **2021**, *384*, 693–704. [CrossRef]
16. Meduri, G.U.; Golden, E.; Freire, A.X.; Taylor, E.; Zaman, M.; Carson, S.J.; Gibson, M.; Umberger, R. Methylprednisolone Infusion in Early Severe ARDS. *Chest* **2007**, *131*, 954–963. [CrossRef]
17. Gupta, S.; Wang, W.; Hayek, S.S.; Chan, L.; Mathews, K.S.; Melamed, M.L.; Brenner, S.K.; Leonberg-Yoo, A.; Schenck, E.J.; Radbel, J.; et al. Association between Early Treatment with Tocilizumab and Mortality among Critically Ill Patients with COVID-19. *JAMA Intern. Med.* **2021**, *181*, 41. [CrossRef]
18. Kaplanski, G.; Bontemps, D.; Esnault, P.; Blasco, V.; Carvelli, J.; Delarbre, D.; Cauchois, R.; Forel, J.-M.; Papazian, L. Combined Anakinra and Ruxolitinib treatment to rescue extremely ill COVID-19 patients: A pilot study. *Autoimmun. Rev.* **2021**, *20*, 102726. [CrossRef]
19. Martin, C.; Brun-Buisson, C. Prise en charge initiale des états septiques graves de l'adulte et de l'enfant. *Réanimation* **2007**, *16*, S1–S21. [CrossRef]
20. Evans, L.; Rhodes, A.; Alhazzani, W.; Antonelli, M.; Coopersmith, C.M.; French, C.; Machado, F.R.; Mcintyre, L.; Ostermann, M.; Prescott, H.C.; et al. Surviving sepsis campaign: International guidelines for management of sepsis and septic shock 2021. *Intensive Care Med.* **2021**, *47*, 1181–1247. [CrossRef]
21. Haute Autorité de Santé. Antibiothérapie des infections à entérobactéries et à Pseudomonas aeruginosa chez l'adulte: Place des carbapénèmes et de leurs alternatives. *Recomm. Bonne Prat.* 2019. Available online: https://www.has-sante.fr/upload/docs/application/pdf/2019-06/synthese_infections_enterobacteries.pdf (accessed on 9 October 2022).
22. Bouadma, L.; Lescure, F.-X.; Lucet, J.-C.; Yazdanpanah, Y.; Timsit, J.-F. Severe SARS-CoV-2 infections: Practical considerations and management strategy for intensivists. *Intensive Care Med.* **2020**, *46*, 579–582. [CrossRef]
23. Tabah, A.; Bassetti, M.; Kollef, M.H.; Zahar, J.-R.; Paiva, J.-A.; Timsit, J.-F.; Roberts, J.A.; Schouten, J.; Giamarellou, H.; Rello, J.; et al. Antimicrobial de-escalation in critically ill patients: A position statement from a task force of the European Society of Intensive Care Medicine (ESICM) and European Society of Clinical Microbiology and Infectious Diseases (ESCMID) Critically Ill Patients Study Group (ESGCIP). *Intensive Care Med.* **2020**, *46*, 245–265. [CrossRef]
24. Fine, J.P.; Gray, R.J. A Proportional Hazards Model for the Subdistribution of a Competing Risk. *J. Am. Stat. Assoc.* **1999**, *94*, 496–509. [CrossRef]
25. Pickens, C.O.; Gao, C.A.; Cuttica, M.J.; Smith, S.B.; Pesce, L.L.; Grant, R.A.; Kang, M.; Morales-Nebreda, L.; Bavishi, A.A.; Arnold, J.M.; et al. Bacterial Superinfection Pneumonia in Patients Mechanically Ventilated for COVID-19 Pneumonia. *Am. J. Respir. Crit. Care Med.* **2021**, *204*, 921–932. [CrossRef]
26. Razazi, K.; Arrestier, R.; Haudebourg, A.F.; Benelli, B.; Carteaux, G.; Decousser, J.; Fourati, S.; Woerther, P.L.; Schlemmer, F.; Charles-Nelson, A.; et al. Risks of ventilator-associated pneumonia and invasive pulmonary aspergillosis in patients with viral acute respiratory distress syndrome related or not to Coronavirus 19 disease. *Crit. Care* **2020**, *24*, 699. [CrossRef]
27. Blonz, G.; Kouatchet, A.; Chudeau, N.; Pontis, E.; Lorber, J.; Lemeur, A.; Planche, L.; Lascarrou, J.-B.; Colin, G. Epidemiology and microbiology of ventilator-associated pneumonia in COVID-19 patients: A multicenter retrospective study in 188 patients in an un-inundated French region. *Crit. Care* **2021**, *25*, 72. [CrossRef]
28. Llitjos, J.-F.; Bredin, S.; Lascarrou, J.-B.; Soumagne, T.; Cojocaru, M.; Leclerc, M.; Lepetit, A.; Gouhier, A.; Charpentier, J.; Piton, G.; et al. Increased susceptibility to intensive care unit-acquired pneumonia in severe COVID-19 patients: A multicentre retrospective cohort study. *Ann. Intensive Care* **2021**, *11*, 20. [CrossRef]
29. The WHO Rapid Evidence Appraisal for COVID-19 Therapies (REACT) Working Group. Association between Administration of IL-6 Antagonists and Mortality among Patients Hospitalized for COVID-19: A Meta-analysis. *JAMA* **2021**, *326*, 499. [CrossRef]
30. Leisman, D.E.; Deutschman, C.S.; Legrand, M. Facing COVID-19 in the ICU: Vascular dysfunction, thrombosis, and dysregulated inflammation. *Intensive Care Med.* **2020**, *46*, 1105–1108. [CrossRef]

31. Ackermann, M.; Verleden, S.E.; Kuehnel, M.; Haverich, A.; Welte, T.; Laenger, F.; Vanstapel, A.; Werlein, C.; Stark, H.; Tzankov, A.; et al. Pulmonary Vascular Endothelialitis, Thrombosis, and Angiogenesis in COVID-19. *N. Engl. J. Med.* **2020**, *383*, 120–128. [CrossRef]
32. Beaucoté, V.; Plantefève, G.; Tirolien, J.-A.; Desaint, P.; Fraissé, M.; Contou, D. Lung Abscess in Critically Ill Coronavirus Disease 2019 Patients with Ventilator-Associated Pneumonia: A French Monocenter Retrospective Study. *Crit. Care Explor.* **2021**, *3*, e0482. [CrossRef]
33. Chastre, J.; Wolff, M.; Fagon, J.-Y.; Chevret, S.; Thomas, F.; Wermert, D.; Clementi, E.; Gonzalez, J.; Jusserand, D.; Asfar, P.; et al. Comparison of 8 vs 15 Days of Antibiotic Therapy for Ventilator-Associated Pneumonia in Adults: A Randomized Trial. *JAMA* **2003**, *290*, 2588. [CrossRef]
34. Chastre, J.; Luyt, C.E. Optimising the duration of antibiotic therapy for ventilator-associated pneumonia. *Eur. Respir. Rev.* **2007**, *16*, 40–44. [CrossRef]
35. Trouillet, J. Les Pneumopathies Acquises Sous Ventilation Mécanique. 2009. Available online: https://sfar.org/les-pneumopathies-acquises-sous-ventilation-mecanique/ (accessed on 9 October 2022).
36. American Thoracic Society; Infectious Diseases Society of America. Guidelines for the Management of Adults with Hospital-acquired, Ventilator-associated, and Healthcare-associated Pneumonia. *Am. J. Respir. Crit. Care Med.* **2005**, *171*, 388–416. [CrossRef]
37. Boumaza, A.; Gay, L.; Mezouar, S.; Bestion, E.; Diallo, A.B.; Michel, M.; Desnues, B.; Raoult, D.; La Scola, B.; Halfon, P.; et al. Monocytes and Macrophages, Targets of Severe Acute Respiratory Syndrome Coronavirus 2: The Clue for Coronavirus Disease 2019 Immunoparalysis. *J. Infect. Dis.* **2021**, *224*, 395–406. [CrossRef]
38. Giacobbe, D.R.; Battaglini, D.; Enrile, E.M.; Dentone, C.; Vena, A.; Robba, C.; Ball, L.; Bartoletti, M.; Coloretti, I.; Di Bella, S.; et al. Incidence and Prognosis of Ventilator-Associated Pneumonia in Critically Ill Patients with COVID-19: A Multicenter Study. *J. Clin. Med.* **2021**, *10*, 555. [CrossRef]
39. Nseir, S.; Martin-Loeches, I.; Povoa, P.; Metzelard, M.; Du Cheyron, D.; Lambiotte, F.; Tamion, F.; Labruyere, M.; Makris, D.; Boulle Geronimi, C.; et al. Relationship between ventilator-associated pneumonia and mortality in COVID-19 patients: A planned ancillary analysis of the coVAPid cohort. *Crit. Care* **2021**, *25*, 177. [CrossRef]

Journal of
Clinical Medicine

MDPI

Article

Effect of the Pandemic Outbreak on ICU-Associated Infections and Antibiotic Prescription Trends in Non-COVID19 Acute Respiratory Failure Patients

Enrico Bussolati [1,†], Rosario Cultrera [1,2,†], Alessandra Quaranta [3], Valentina Cricca [3], Elisabetta Marangoni [3], Riccardo La Rosa [1], Sara Bertacchini [3], Alessandra Bellonzi [3], Riccardo Ragazzi [1,3], Carlo Alberto Volta [1,3], Savino Spadaro [1,3] and Gaetano Scaramuzzo [1,3,*]

1 Department of Translational Medicine, University of Ferrara, 44121 Ferrara, Italy
2 Infectious Diseases Unit, Azienda Ospedaliera Universitaria Sant'Anna, 44121 Ferrara, Italy
3 Intensive Care Unit, Azienda Ospedaliera Universitaria Sant'Anna, 44121 Ferrara, Italy
* Correspondence: scrgtn@unife.it
† These authors contributed equally to this work.

Abstract: Background: The COVID-19 pandemic had a relevant impact on the organization of intensive care units (ICU) and may have reduced the overall compliance with healthcare-associated infections (HAIs) prevention programs. Invasively ventilated patients are at high risk of ICU-associated infection, but there is little evidence regarding the impact of the pandemic on their occurrence in non-COVID-19 patients. Moreover, little is known of antibiotic prescription trends in the ICU during the first wave of the pandemic. The purpose of this investigation is to assess the incidence, characteristics, and risk factors for ICU-associated HAIs in a population of invasively ventilated patients affected by non-COVID-19 acute respiratory failure (ARF) admitted to the ICU in the first wave of the COVID-19 pandemic, and to evaluate the ICU antimicrobial prescription strategies. Moreover, we compared HAIs and antibiotic use to a cohort of ARF patients admitted to the ICU the year before the pandemic during the same period. Methods: this is a retrospective, single-centered cohort study conducted at S. Anna University Hospital (Ferrara, Italy). We enrolled patients admitted to the ICU for acute respiratory failure requiring invasive mechanical ventilation (MV) between February and April 2020 (intra-pandemic group, IP) and February and April 2019 (before the pandemic group, PP). We excluded patients admitted to the ICU for COVID-19 pneumonia. We recorded patients' baseline characteristics, ICU-associated procedures and devices. Moreover, we evaluated antimicrobial therapy and classified it as prophylactic, empirical or target therapy, according to the evidence of infection at the time of prescription and to the presence of a positive culture sample. We compared the results of the two groups (PP and IP) to assess differences between the two years. Results: One hundred and twenty-eight patients were screened for inclusion and 83 patients were analyzed, 45 and 38 in the PP and I group, respectively. We found a comparable incidence of HAIs (62.2% vs. 65.8%, $p = 0.74$) and multidrug-resistant (MDR) isolations (44.4% vs. 36.8% $p = 0.48$) in the two groups. The year of ICU admission was not independently associated with an increased risk of developing HAIs (OR = 0.35, 95% CI 0.16–1.92, $p = 0.55$). The approach to antimicrobial therapy was characterized by a significant reduction in total antimicrobial use (21.4 ± 18.7 vs. 11.6 ± 9.4 days, $p = 0.003$), especially of target therapy, in the IP group. Conclusions: ICU admission for non-COVID-19 ARF during the first wave of the SARS-CoV-2 pandemic was not associated with an increased risk of ICU-associated HAIs. Nevertheless, ICU prescription of antimicrobial therapy changed and significantly decreased during the pandemic.

Keywords: healthcare-associated infections; multidrug resistance; COVID-19; acute respiratory failure; mechanical ventilation; antimicrobial therapy; SARS-CoV-2 pandemic1

Citation: Bussolati, E.; Cultrera, R.; Quaranta, A.; Cricca, V.; Marangoni, E.; La Rosa, R.; Bertacchini, S.; Bellonzi, A.; Ragazzi, R.; Volta, C.A.; et al. Effect of the Pandemic Outbreak on ICU-Associated Infections and Antibiotic Prescription Trends in Non-COVID19 Acute Respiratory Failure Patients. *J. Clin. Med.* **2022**, *11*, 7080. https://doi.org/10.3390/jcm11237080

Academic Editor: Michael Dreher

Received: 8 November 2022
Accepted: 25 November 2022
Published: 29 November 2022

1. Introduction

Healthcare-associated infections (HAIs) and HAIs-related septic shock are the leading causes of death in noncardiac intensive care units (ICUs) and, despite advances in modern intensive care, their incidence is still rising [1]. Several factors are associated with the increase in HAIs, such as patients' comorbidities, increased use of invasive devices, long-lasting antibiotic therapies and frequent contact with healthcare personnel caring for multiple patients [2–4].

The SARS-CoV-2 pandemic outbreak had an enormous impact on worldwide health, causing over 533 million confirmed cases and over 6.3 million deaths worldwide by 12 June 2022 (according to the WHO Coronavirus disease situation report). Up to 25% of infected patients were admitted to an ICU, 80% of them requiring invasive mechanical ventilation (MV) [5,6]. The magnitude of the coronavirus disease 2019 (COVID-19) pandemic required the reorganization of healthcare facilities, concerning both the increase of ICUs beds and the improvement in human and material resources. These "new" ICUs were characterized by the extensive use of personal protective equipment (PPE), increased workload and by the presence of healthcare professionals deployed from other areas [7]. All these reasons may have reduced the overall compliance with HAI prevention programs, independently of COVID-19 infection [8,9].

Although the incidence of HAIs in the COVID-19 population has been extensively studied [10–15], the indirect effect of the pandemic on the occurrence of HAIs in non-COVID-19 acute respiratory failure patients is still unknown. An association between hospitalization during the pandemic and HAIs was found in patients admitted to the neurology ward and stroke units [16], but the impact of the pandemic on HAIs in ICU non-COVID-19 ARF patients remains unknown.

Moreover, despite few data demonstrating an overall reduction in antibiotic use in outreach patients, little is known regarding the ICU antimicrobial prescription trends during the first wave of the COVID-19 pandemic.

We therefore hypothesized that the pandemic could have had indirect effects on ICU antimicrobial prescription trends and on the incidence and characteristics of ICU-associated HAIs, especially in the first wave of the pandemic.

To test this hypothesis, we assessed the incidence, characteristics and risk factors for HAIs and the ICU antimicrobial management of patients admitted to the ICU for non-COVID-19 acute respiratory failure requiring invasive mechanical ventilation during the first wave of the COVID-19 pandemic (February–April 2020). Furthermore, we compared this group to patients admitted to the same ICU during the same period in the year before the pandemic (February–April 2019).

2. Materials and Methods

2.1. Study Population and Protocol

This is a retrospective, single-center, observational cohort study of patients admitted to the ICU of the S. Anna University Hospital (Ferrara, Italy) over a period of 3 months (February, March and April) of two consecutive years, before (2019) and during the first wave (2020) of the COVID-19 pandemic. The first wave of the pandemic was defined as the time from the first detected case (31 January 2020) to the start of reopening after the national lockdown (26 April 2020). The study was approved by the institutional ethics board of Area Vasta Emilia Centrale, site in IRCCS Azienda Ospedaliera—Universitaria di Bologna, Policlinico S. Orsola-Malpighi (Protocol number 235/2022/Oss/AOUFe), and informed consent was collected or waived if collection was not possible according to the local regulations.

2.2. Inclusions and Exclusions Criteria

All consecutive patients admitted to the ICU during the study period were screened for inclusion. The inclusion criteria were: age 18–90 years; invasive mechanical ventilation; ICU admission for acute respiratory failure requiring invasive mechanical ventilation;

and availability of a digital clinical record with detailed information on therapy and devices used during ICU stay. Exclusion criteria were: incomplete or incorrect records; unavailability of cultural samples data during ICU stay; presence of positive cultural isolations on admission and ICU admission for COVID-19-related acute respiratory failure.

2.3. Study Protocol and Definitions

For all patients admitted to the ICU and meeting inclusion criteria, data about demographics (i.e., age, sex, height, weight), comorbidities, ICU entrance diagnosis, medication before ICU admission, the Simplified Acute Physiology Score (SAPS) II, which is an index of disease severity [17], and duration of hospital stay before ICU admission were collected.

We collected data on ventilatory features (duration of invasive and non-invasive ventilation, oxygen therapy, tracheostomy and eventually prone positioning), invasive device features (central venous line, midline and arterial line), and presence and duration of laparostomy. Ventilatory free days (VFDs) were calculated as previously described [18]. As concerns antimicrobial therapy, we defined it as prophylactic, empiric or target according to the evidence of infection when the antimicrobial treatment was started. Specifically, we defined as (1) prophylactic any antimicrobial therapy prescribed in the absence of any sign and symptom of infection (e.g., fever, leukocytosis, increase of PCR/procalcitonin); as (2) empiric any therapy initiated without any positive cultural isolation in presence of signs and/or symptoms of infection; and as (3) target any therapy started after positive cultural isolation.

We also defined days on antimicrobial therapy as the number of days on antimicrobial treatment, independently of how many drugs were prescribed at the same time. Total antimicrobial use was defined as the cumulative sum of days on therapy for all antimicrobials during ICU stay, as previously defined by Campbell et al. [19]. Outcomes regarding length of ICU stay, mortality, microbiologic isolations (bloodstream, respiratory tract and urinary tract cultures) and multidrug resistance were also collected.

We defined HAIs as infections acquired at least 48 h after ICU admission. Bloodstream, respiratory tract and urinary tract microbial identification, antimicrobial susceptibility, multidrug resistance and MIC interpretation were defined as previously described by Cultrera et al. [10]. The isolations referring to blood, respiratory and urine cultures were requested by the attending physicians for patients with suspected secondary infections because of clinical and/or respiratory deterioration associated with suggestive laboratory or radiological findings.

2.4. Statistical Analyses

Categorical variables are reported as frequency, while continuous variables as mean $\pm$ standard deviation or median [interquartile range], according to data distribution (normal/not normal). Considering the absence of evidence regarding HAIs in non-COVID-19 patients during the first wave of the COVID-19 pandemic, we could not calculate a priori the sample size and therefore aimed to enroll the higher number of patients admitted to the ICU during the study period. Patients were assigned to one of the groups (PP and IP) based on the year of ICU admission.

Bivariate comparisons regarding nominal data were conducted using Pearson's chi-square test. The Shapiro–Wilk test was used to verify continuous variables distribution. Student's t-test and Mann–Whitney U test were used to compare the two samples (depending on normality distribution). Logistic regression technique was performed to evaluate risk factors associated with HAIs, and the outcome was defined as presence/absence of HAIs during ICU stay. The predictors inserted in the regression model were: the year of admission, positive history of Diabetes Mellitus, Chronic Kidney Disease (CKD), smoking, obesity (defined as BMI > 30), ICU length of stay, duration of invasive mechanical ventilation and duration of steroid therapy.

A linear multiple regression was used to test the association of SAPS II, presence of heart diseases, lung diseases, DM, CKD, year of ICU admission, duration of ICU stay, duration IMV and admission to the ICU after surgery with total antimicrobial use. Significance was set at $p < 0.05$. Statistical Analysis was performed using SPSS 24 (IBM Corp. Released 2016. IBM SPSS Statistics for Windows, Version 24.0. IBM Corp, Armonk, NY, USA) and GraphPad Prism version 8.0.0 for Windows (GraphPad Software, San Diego, CA, USA, www.graphpad.com, accessed on 1 June 2022).

3. Results

3.1. Baseline Population Characteristics

Figure 1 describes the patient selection process. Two-hundred and eleven patients were admitted to the ICU during the study period and screened for inclusion. After evaluating for inclusion and exclusion criteria, a total of 83 patients were included in the study. Their main clinical characteristics are described in Table 1.

Table 1. Baseline characteristics at ICU admission, comorbidities, and entrance diagnosis.

Parameter	PP, n = 45	IP, n = 38	p Value
Age (years)	71.4 ± 14.1	70.16 ± 10.5	0.66
Females (number)	18 (40%)	18 (47.4%)	0.50
Weight (kg)	75.7 ± 20.1	79.8 ± 16.1	0.32
Height (cm)	168.6 ± 10	168.5 ± 7.3	0.98
BMI (kg/m2)	26.5 ± 5.5	28.1 ± 5.7	0.19
Hypertension (yes)	32 (71.1%)	28 (73.7%)	0.79
Heart Disease (yes)	25 (55.6%)	13 (34.2%)	0.052
Pneumopathy (yes)	13 (28.9%)	9 (23.7%)	0.59
CKD (yes)	13 (28.9%)	3 (7.9%)	*0.016*
DM (yes)	10 (22.2%)	11 (28.9%)	0.48
Immunosuppression (yes)	7 (15.6%)	5 (13.2%)	0.76
SAPS II	47 ± 17.7	48.1 ± 16.5	0.77
Hospital stay before ICU (days)	4.1 ± 7	6.8 ± 26.3	0.52
Smoke			0.89
Current smokers	8 (22.2%)	7 (18.4%)	
Former smokers	9 (25%)	11 (28.9%)	
Reasons for ICU amission			0.35
Acute respiratory failure after surgery	25 (55.6%)	19 (50%)	
Septic Shock	4 (8.9%)	10 (26.3%)	
Pneumopathy	8 (17.8%)	3 (7.9%)	
Neuropathy	4 (8.9%)	2 (5.3%)	
Trauma	2 (4.4%)	2 (5.3%)	
Heart Disease	1 (2.2%)	1 (2.6%)	
Metabolic Disease	1 (2.2%)	0 (0%)	
Other	0 (0%)	1 (2.6%)	

Data are expressed as Mean ± SMean SD or Number (%), according to the data. PP, pre-pandemic; IP, intra-pandemic; BMI, Body mass index; CKD, chronic kidney disease; DM, diabetes mellitus; SAPS II, Simplified Acute Physiology Score II. Italic for categories.

When comparing the PP and the IP groups, the mean age of the two groups was comparable (Table 1). No significant differences were observed either in anthropometric parameters or comorbidities, with the sole exception of chronic kidney disease ($p = 0.016$). No significant differences were seen in the ICU entrance diagnosis ($p = 0.35$) and in the duration of hospital stay before ICU ($p = 0.52$, Table 1).

3.2. Clinical Features

The clinical characteristics during the ICU stay are resumed in Table 2. ICU length of stay ($p = 0.92$), ICU mortality ($p = 0.68$), the duration of invasive ventilation ($p = 0.41$), VFDs ($p = 0.12$) and the number of patients undergoing non-invasive ventilation, oxygen therapy, tracheostomy and pronation were not different between the two groups.

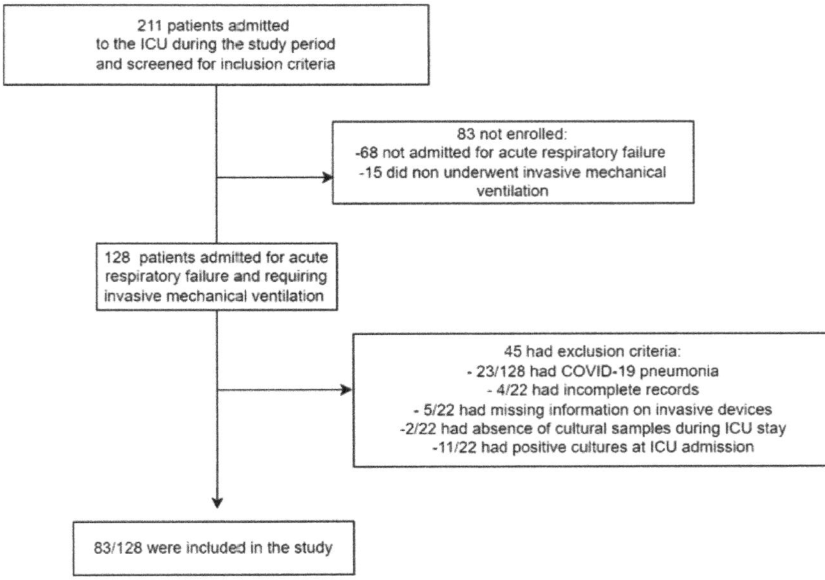

Figure 1. Flow diagram of patient selection process.

Table 2. Clinical features (outcomes, therapies, ventilatory, catheter and others) during ICU stay.

Parameter	PP, n = 45	IP, n = 38	p Value
ICU length of stay (days)	7.7 ± 8	7.6 ± 5.9	0.92
Dead during ICU (yes)	9 (20%)	9 (23.7%)	0.68
Duration of Invasive Ventilation (days)	4.3 ± 5.5	5.2 ± 4.7	0.41
Ventilatory Free Days (days)	24 [19.5–27]	21.5 [7.5–26.2]	0.12
Non-Invasive Ventilation (yes)	2 (4.4%)	2 (5.3%)	0.86
Oxygen therapy (yes)	34 (75.6%)	28 (73.7%)	0.84
Tracheostomy (yes)	6 (13.3%)	2 (5.3%)	0.21
Prone positioning (yes)	1 (2.3)	1 (2.6)	0.92
Catheter Features			
Patients with central venous line	42 (93%)	38 (100%)	0.10
Patients with midline	2 (4.4%)	0 (0%)	0.19
Patients with arterial line	44 (97.8 %)	35 (92.1%)	0.23
Central venous lines/patient during ICU stay	1 [1,2]	1 [1,2]	0.41
Site of first CVC cannulation			0.08
Subclavian	2 (4.4%)	3 (7.9%)	
Jugular	36 (80%)	35 (92.1%)	
Femoral	4 (8.9%)	0 (0%)	
Presence of laparostomy (yes)	3 (6.7%)	5 (13.2%)	0.32
Duration of laparostomy (Days)	5 ± 4.6	2.6 ± 1.5	0.46
Steroid Therapy during ICU stay (nr. of patients)	30 (66.7%)	22 (57.9%)	0.41
Duration of Steroid Therapy during ICU stay (days)	7.5 ± 12.3	3.1 ± 5.8	*0.038*
Total Steroid Dosage (mg Hydrocortisone/kg)	16.3 ± 31.1	14.4 ± 38	0.81
Vasoactive drugs > 0.1 γ/Kg/min (number of patients)	26 (57.8%)	27 (71.1%)	0.21

Data are expressed as Mean ± SD, Median [IQR] or Number (%), according to the data. PP, pre-pandemic; IP, intra-pandemic; CVC, central venous catheter. Italic for categories.

A similar number of patients between the two groups had a central venous line, a midline and/or an arterial line. In the IP group, no patient had a first central venous line inserted at the femoral site, consequently resulting in an increased number of jugular and subclavian insertion sites, although this did not reach statistical significance. The duration of steroid therapy was significantly shorter in the IP group (7.5 ± 12.3 days (PP) and 3.1 ± 5.8 (IP) (p = 0.038)).

3.3. Antimicrobial Therapy

In the IP group, the total antimicrobial use was significantly shorter (11.6 ± 9.4 days) than in the PP group (21.4 ± 18.7 days, p = 0.003), while the days on antimicrobial therapy were similar between the groups (6.6 ± 5.2 vs. 6.6 ± 4.2, p = 0.97, Table 3). The year of ICU stay was also independently associated with total antimicrobial use when adjusting for possible confounders in the regression model (Std. Beta 0.280, p = 0.003, Table S1). The duration of 2nd and 3rd antimicrobials were significantly shorter in terms of days in the IP group (p = 0.037 and p = 0.019, respectively).

Table 3. Antimicrobial therapy, cultural samples and infections in the study population, divided for year of admission.

Parameter	PP, n = 45	IP, n = 38	p Value
Total antimicrobial use (days)	21.4 ± 18.7	11.6 ± 9.4	*0.003*
Day on antimicrobial therapy (days)	6.6 ± 5.2	6.64 ± 4.2	0.97
Number of different antimicrobials/patients	2.67 ± 1.6	2.22 ± 1.2	0.16
Duration of 1st Antimicrobial (days)	6.7 ± 4.8	5.3 ± 3.7	0.13
Duration of 2nd Antimicrobial (days)	5.3 ± 5.4	3.3 ± 3.3	*0.037*
Duration of 3rd Antimicrobial (days)	4.9 ± 7.6	1.9 ± 3.3	*0.019*
Patients with HAIs	28 (62.2%)	25 (65.8%)	0.74
Cultural samples per patient	8.24 ± 7.8	7.84 ± 6.2	0.79
Positive cultural samples per patient	1 [0–2.5]	1 [0–3.2]	0.50
Patients with an MDR infection	20 (44.4%)	14 (36.8%)	0.48
MDR positive isolations/patient	0 [0–1]	0 [0–1]	0.52
Patients with MDR bloodstream infections	12 (26.7%)	8 (21.1%)	0.55
Patients with MDR respiratory infections	13 (28.9%)	7 (18.4%)	0.27
Patients with MDR urinary infections	1 (2.2%)	1 (2.6%)	0.90

Data are expressed as Mean ± SD, Median [IQR] or Number (%), according to the data. PP, pre-pandemic; IP, intra-pandemic; MDR, multidrug-resistant.

A higher number of patients underwent prophylactic therapy (p = 0.03) and a lower number of patients underwent empiric therapy (p = 0.05) in the PP group (Figure 2). Despite this, the number of days for each therapy was not significantly different, except for target therapy, which decreased from PP to IP (p = 0.03). No significative differences could be found between the groups in the antimicrobial class prescription. Nevertheless, there was a tendency towards an increased prescription of Penicillin and Carbapenems and a decreased prescription of antifungals (Figure 3).

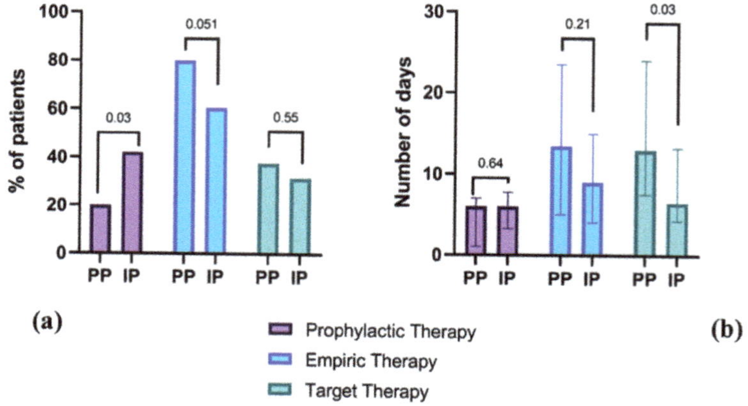

Figure 2. Comparison of different antimicrobial approaches before and during the pandemic. (**a**) Percentage of patients who underwent prophylactic, empiric and target therapy in the two study populations; (**b**) Number of days undergoing prophylactic, empiric and target therapy in the two years of analysis, i.e., pre-pandemic (2019) and intra-pandemic (2020). PP, pre-pandemic; IP, intra-pandemic.

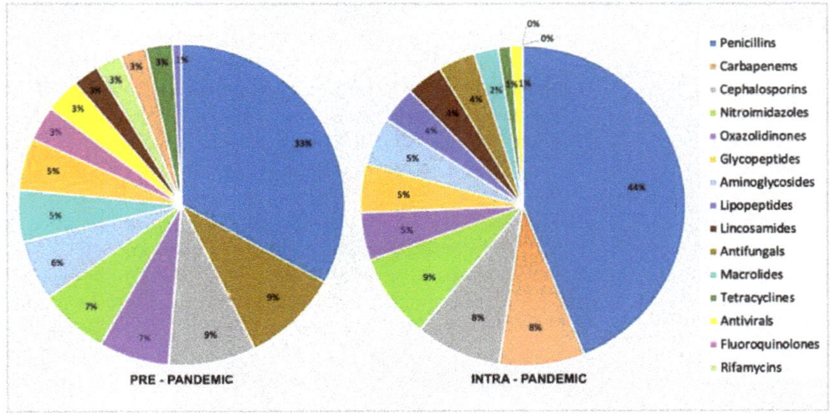

Figure 3. Antimicrobial classes and relative percentages regarding every administered drug in the two years of analysis (pre-Pandemic and intra-pandemic).

3.4. Cultural Isolations

There were no significant differences between the two groups in the number of cultural samples/patient, positive cultural samples/patient and number of patients developing HAIs and MDR infections, as shown in Table 3. Microbial isolations in blood, respiratory tract and urinary tract were divided in families and differences are summarized in Table S2 and Figure S1. The only significant difference between PP and IP was the increased number of *Candida* spp. isolations ($p < 0.001$) in the IP group, mostly isolated from the respiratory and urinary tract.

3.5. Multivariate Analysis

The multivariate logistic regression analysis on risk factors associated with HAIs is shown in Table 4. In the analysis, only CKD was significantly associated with HAIs ($p = 0.024$), while being admitted to the ICU during the pandemic was not.

Table 4. Multivariate logistic regression analysis on risk factors associated with healthcare-associated infections, with outcome defined as presence/absence of HAIs during ICU stay.

	Multivariate Analysis			
	OR	Sig.	95% C.I. for OR	
			Lower	Upper
Year of admission (IP)	0.35	0.55	0.16	1.92
DM (yes)	0.65	0.53	0.17	2.50
CKD (yes)	14.40	0.024	1.43	146.26
Smoke (yes)	0.41	0.30	0.08	2.23
Former smokers (yes)	0.98	0.98	0.24	4.06
Tracheostomy (yes)	3.47	0.35	0.25	47.71
Obesity (yes)	0.50	0.31	0.13	1.95
ICU stay (days)	1.10	0.31	0.91	1.33
IMV duration (days)	1.22	0.09	0.97	1.55
Steroid therapy (days)	1.03	0.55	0.94	1.13

Reference in parenthesis; IP, Intra-Pandemic (2020); CKD, chronic kidney disease; DM, diabetes mellitus; ICU, intensive care unit; IMV, invasive mechanical ventilation.

4. Discussion

In this study, ICU admission for non-COVID-19 acute respiratory failure requiring invasive mechanical ventilation during the first wave of the COVID-19 pandemic was not associated with an increased risk of healthcare-associated infection. As concerns multidrug resistance, no difference was observed in the number of patients developing MDR infections, neither considering cumulative cultures, nor respectively comparing bloodstream, respiratory tract, and urinary tract infections. Finally, we observed a change into the approach to the antimicrobial therapy, with an increased attention to antibiotic de-escalation and a lower total antimicrobial use.

Several studies explored the epidemiology of ICU infections during the COVID-19 pandemic. The overall increased incidence of HAIs reported during the pandemic [11] could be related to environmental causes (new ICU beds in other spaces in the hospital or ICU, incorporation of new doctors and nurses not previously trained in critical care, changes in the standards of patient care, use of PPI during long shifts) [12] or to the immunological and/or therapeutic characteristics of the COVID-19 infection [13]. Although HAIs in COVID-19 patients are increased [14,15], the relative role of the environmental and/or disease related factors is still not clear. By analyzing non-COVID-19 patients, we found that HAI incidence did not increase during the first wave of the pandemic. Therefore, the increased risk of HAIs already previously found in COVID-19 patients, as compared to non-COVID-19 patients [11,20], may be related to the immunological dysregulation determined by the SARS-CoV-2 virus [21] and/or to use of immunomodulatory drugs [22,23], more than it is related to environmental reasons.

Baccolini et al. [11] observed a higher proportion of HAIs in COVID-19 patients, compared to non-COVID-19 patients (admitted both before and during pandemic), but did not compare HAIs between non-COVID-19 patients admitted before and during the pandemic. They hypothesized a relation between better outcomes in non-COVID-19 patients and a less severe clinical situation on admission during the pandemic, due to social lock-down measures and fear of becoming infected inside the hospitals. Shbaklo et al. [24] observed a reduction in MDR infections during the first wave of the COVID-19 pandemic (the same period as our observation) compared with an increase in the overall bacterial infections during the late period of the pandemic. They attributed this to the growing adherence to infection prevention and control (IPC) procedures [25–27], suggesting that the COVID-19 pandemic may have raised awareness of the need to prevent HAIs and increased the compliance of healthcare workers to IPC in the ICU. We can confirm these findings as we found a comparable incidence of ICU HAIs before and after the start of the COVID-19 pandemic. Moreover, we found no difference in the simplified acute physiology score II (SAPS II) and in diagnosis on admission that were therefore comparable in gravity.

We also assessed the effect of the pandemic on the approach to antimicrobial therapy in ICU patients with ARF. The antimicrobial approach is determined by antimicrobial stewardship programs, listing among the objectives the sustainability of empirical and target treatments (performed through antibiotic selection), dose adjustments, drug monitoring de-escalation and shortening duration to reduce multidrug resistance and selective pressure [28]. We found that being admitted to the ICU in the before the pandemic period was independently associated with a higher risk of antimicrobial use (Table S1). Despite this, we observed no difference in the duration of ICU stay, mortality and number of MDR infections after the shortening of both overall antimicrobial and target therapy in the IP group, as confirmed by previous evidence [29].

Our findings on the tendency to reduced antimicrobial use during the pandemic are in line with the data of the European Centre for Disease Prevention and Control (ECDC), which showed a decrease in the total antibiotic consumption in humans between 2019 and 2020 in both community [30] and hospital settings [31]. Although the report does not provide definite reasons for the reduction in antimicrobial prescription, the reasons may be found in the increase in ICU-related antimicrobial stewardship programs [32] and probably in the redistribution of resources for the ongoing pandemic, which led to a stricter tendency in antibiotic prescription. Interestingly, we also reported a decrease in the duration of steroid therapy during the first wave of the pandemic. Although the cumulative dose was not different among groups, the therapy was shorter in the IP group. This may also be connected to a higher awareness of the side effects of prolonged steroid therapy on HAIs and therefore is strongly linked to our findings on antibiotic prescription trends. Nevertheless, although the duration of steroid therapy was different, it was not associated with changes in HAI incidence. This could also be an issue considering the possible link between corticosteroid therapy and HAIs previously reported for COVID-19 patients [33].

When analyzing the microbial species associated with HAIs, it was found that *Candida* spp. was the only microorganism whose percentage of isolation increased between PP and IP, becoming the most frequently isolated family of the IP group. Fungal deaths increased during 2020–2021 compared with previous years, primarily driven by COVID-19, particularly those involving *Aspergillus* spp. and *Candida* spp. [34]. Poor data are available on non-COVID-19 patients admitted during the pandemic. Interestingly, the increase of *Candida* spp. infections did not seem to affect the duration of ICU stay, MV and mortality.

Our study has some limitations. First, it is a retrospective single-center cohort study evaluating a limited number of patients. Secondly, the classification of antimicrobial therapy was conducted a posteriori by analyzing the medical records. Thirdly, since the number of patients enrolled in our study is limited, the results must be considered exploratory. Finally, we only evaluated a limited period during the COVID-19 pandemic. Since some recommendations regarding antibiotic prescription changed over time [35], our findings refers only to the first wave of the pandemic and cannot be applied to the other periods.

5. Conclusions

ICU admission during the first wave of the COVID-19 pandemic for non-COVID-19 acute respiratory failure was not associated with a higher risk of developing hospital-associated infections. The first wave of the pandemic was characterized by an overall reduction in antimicrobial use in non-COVID-19 patients. Furthermore, this reduction was not related to an increase in hospital-acquired infections or to a worsening of ICU outcomes.

Supplementary Materials: The following supporting information can be downloaded at: https://www.mdpi.com/article/10.3390/jcm11237080/s1, Figure S1: Relative percentage of isolated microorganisms' classes in the cumulative positive cultures, bloodstream cultures, respiratory tract cultures and urinary tract cultures in the two years of analysis. PP, pre-pandemic; IP, intra-pandemic.; Table S1: Multivariate Analysis on risk factors associated to total antimicrobial use; Table S2: Microbial isolations in blood, respiratory tract and urinary tract samples, divided in families in the two years.

Author Contributions: Conceptualization: R.C., C.A.V., S.S. and G.S.; Data curation, E.B., A.Q. and G.S.; Formal analysis, E.B. and G.S.; Investigation, A.Q.; Methodology, S.S.; Resources, E.M. and R.R.; Supervision, R.C., E.M., S.B., A.B., R.R. and G.S.; Visualization, V.C. and C.A.V.; Writing—original draft, E.B.; Writing—review and editing, R.C., V.C., R.L.R., C.A.V., S.S. and G.S. All authors have read and agreed to the published version of the manuscript.

Funding: This research received no external funding.

Institutional Review Board Statement: The study was conducted in accordance with the Declaration of Helsinki, and approved by the Ethics Committee of Area Vasta Emilia Centro (IRCCS Azienda Ospedaliera—Universitaria di Bologna, Policlinico S. Orsola-Malpighi; Protocol number 235/2022/Oss/AOUFe, date of approval 18 May 2022).

Informed Consent Statement: Informed consent was obtained or waived when collection was not possible due to the retrospective nature of the analysis, according to local regulations.

Data Availability Statement: The data presented in this study are available on request from the corresponding author.

Acknowledgments: We would like to thank the staff of the Azienda Ospedaliera Universitaria of Ferrara who collaborated in the clinical management of the patients, especially during the pandemic.

Conflicts of Interest: The authors declare no conflict of interest.

References

1. Vincent, J.; Rello, J.; Marshall, J.; Silva, E.; Anzueto, A.; Martin, C.D.; Moreno, R.; Lipman, J.; Gomersall, C.; Sakr, Y.; et al. International study of the prevalence and outcomes of infection in intensive care units. *JAMA* **2009**, *302*, 2323–2329. [CrossRef] [PubMed]
2. Hynes-Gay, P.; Lalla, P.; Leo, M.; Merrill-Bell, A.; Nicholson, M.; Villaruel, E. Understanding sepsis: From SIRS to septic shock. *Dynamics* **2002**, *13*, 17–20, 22–24; quiz 25–26. [PubMed]
3. Kaye, K.S.; Marchaim, O.; Smialowicz, C.; Bentley, L. Suction Regulators: A Potential Vector for Hospital-Acquired Pathogens. *Infect. Control Hosp. Epidemiol.* **2010**, *31*, 772–774. [CrossRef] [PubMed]
4. Bonten, M.J. Colonization pressure: A critical parameter in the epidemiology of antibiotic-resistant bacteria. *Crit. Care* **2012**, *16*, 142. [CrossRef] [PubMed]
5. Wang, D.; Hu, B.; Hu, C.; Zhu, F.; Liu, X.; Zhang, J.; Wang, B.; Xiang, H.; Cheng, Z.; Xiong, Y.; et al. Clinical Characteristics of 138 Hospitalized Patients With 2019 Novel Coronavirus—Infected Pneumonia in Wuhan, China. *JAMA* **2020**, *323*, 1061–1069. [CrossRef]
6. Grasselli, G.; Zangrillo, A.; Zanella, A.; Antonelli, M.; Cabrini, L.; Castelli, A.; Cereda, D.; Coluccello, A.; Foti, G.; Fumagalli, R.; et al. Baseline Characteristics and Outcomes of 1591 Patients Infected With SARS-CoV-2 Admitted to ICUs of the Lombardy Region, Italy. *JAMA* **2020**, *323*, 1574–1581, Erratum in *JAMA* **2021**, *325*, 2120. [CrossRef]
7. El-Hage, W.; Hingray, C.; Lemogne, C.; Yrondi, A.; Brunault, P.; Bienvenu, T.; Etain, B.; Paquet, C.; Gohier, B.; Bennabi, D.; et al. Health professionals facing the coronavirus disease 2019 (COVID-19) pandemic: What are the mental health risks? *Encephale* **2020**, *46*, S73–S80. [CrossRef]
8. Blot, S.; Ruppé, E.; Harbarth, S.; Asehnoune, K.; Poulakou, G.; Luyt, C.-E.; Rello, J.; Klompas, M.; Depuydt, P.; Eckmann, C.; et al. Healthcare-associated infections in adult intensive care unit patients: Changes in epidemiology, diagnosis, prevention and contributions of new technologies. *Intensive Crit. Care Nurs.* **2022**, *70*, 103227. [CrossRef]
9. Fakih, M.G.; Bufalino, A.; Sturm, L.; Huang, R.-H.; Ottenbacher, A.; Saake, K.; Winegar, A.; Fogel, R.; Cacchione, J. Coronavirus disease 2019 (COVID-19) pandemic, central-line–associated bloodstream infection (CLABSI), and catheter-associated urinary tract infection (CAUTI): The urgent need to refocus on hardwiring prevention efforts. *Infect. Control. Hosp. Epidemiology* **2021**, *43*, 26–31. [CrossRef]
10. Cultrera, R.; Barozzi, A.; Libanore, M.; Marangoni, E.; Pora, R.; Quarta, B.; Spadaro, S.; Ragazzi, R.; Marra, A.; Segala, D.; et al. Co-Infections in Critically Ill Patients with or without COVID-19: A Comparison of Clinical Microbial Culture Findings. *Int. J. Environ. Res. Public Health* **2021**, *18*, 4358. [CrossRef]
11. Baccolini, V.; Migliara, G.; Isonne, C.; Dorelli, B.; Barone, L.C.; Giannini, D.; Marotta, D.; Marte, M.; Mazzalai, E.; Alessandri, F.; et al. The impact of the COVID-19 pandemic on healthcare-associated infections in intensive care unit patients: A retrospective cohort study. *Antimicrob. Resist. Infect. Control.* **2021**, *10*, 87. [CrossRef] [PubMed]
12. Marin-Corral, J.; Pascual-Guardia, S.; Muñoz-Bermúdez, R.; Salazar-Degracia, A.; Climent, C.; Vilà-Vilardell, C.; Acer, M.; Picornell, M.; Restrepo, M.; Masclans, J.; et al. Health care-associated infections in patients with COVID-19 pneumonia in COVID critical care areas. *Med. Intensiv.* **2021**, *46*, 221–223. [CrossRef] [PubMed]
13. Chen, G.; Wu, D.; Guo, W.; Cao, Y.; Huang, D.; Wang, H.; Wang, T.; Zhang, X.; Chen, H.; Yu, H.; et al. Clinical and immunological features of severe and moderate coronavirus disease 2019. *J. Clin. Investig.* **2020**, *130*, 2620–2629. [CrossRef] [PubMed]
14. Grasselli, G.; Scaravilli, V.; Mangioni, D.; Scudeller, L.; Alagna, L.; Bartoletti, M.; Bellani, G.; Biagioni, E.; Bonfanti, P.; Bottino, N.; et al. Hospital-Acquired Infections in Critically Ill Patients With COVID-19. *Chest* **2021**, *160*, 454–465. [CrossRef] [PubMed]
15. Smith, L.; Karaba, S.M.; Amoah, J.; Jones, G.; Avery, R.K.; Dzintars, K.; Helsel, T.; Cosgrove, S.E.; Fabre, V. Hospital-acquired infections among adult patients admitted for coronavirus disease 2019 (COVID-19). *Infect. Control Hosp. Epidemiol.* **2021**, *43*, 1054–1057. [CrossRef]
16. Cerulli Irelli, E.; Orlando, B.; Cocchi, E.; Morano, A.; Fattapposta, F.; Di Piero, V.; Toni, D.; Ciardi, M.R.; Giallonardo, A.T.; Fabbrini, G.; et al. The potential impact of enhanced hygienic measures during the COVID-19 outbreak on hospital-acquired infections: A pragmatic study in neurological units. *J. Neurol. Sci.* **2020**, *418*, 117111. [CrossRef]
17. Le Gall, J.R.; Lemeshow, S.; Saulnier, F. A new Simplified Acute Physiology Score (SAPS II) based on a European/North American multicenter study. *JAMA* **1993**, *270*, 2957–2963. [CrossRef]
18. Schoenfeld, D.A.; Bernard, G.R. Statistical evaluation of ventilator-free days as an efficacy measure in clinical trials of treatments for acute respiratory distress syndrome. *Crit. Care Med.* **2002**, *30*, 1772–1777. [CrossRef]
19. Campbell, T.J.; Decloe, M.; Gill, S.; Ho, G.; McCready, J.; Powis, J. Every antibiotic, every day: Maximizing the impact of prospective audit and feedback on total antibiotic use. *PLoS ONE* **2017**, *12*, e0178434. [CrossRef]
20. Buetti, N.; Ruckly, S.; de Montmollin, E.; Reignier, J.; Terzi, N.; Cohen, Y.; Siami, S.; Dupuis, C.; Timsit, J.-F. COVID-19 increased the risk of ICU-acquired bloodstream infections: A case–cohort study from the multicentric OUTCOMEREA network. *Intensive Care Med.* **2021**, *47*, 180–187. [CrossRef]
21. Parrill, A.; Tsao, T.; Dong, V.; Huy, N.T. SARS-CoV-2-induced immunodysregulation and the need for higher clinical suspicion for co-infection and secondary infection in COVID-19 patients. *J. Microbiol. Immunol. Infect.* **2020**, *54*, 105–108. [CrossRef]
22. Pawar, A.; Desai, R.J.; Solomon, D.H.; Ortiz, A.J.S.; Gale, S.; Bao, M.; Sarsour, K.; Schneeweiss, S.; Kim, S.C. Risk of serious infections in tocilizumab versus other biologic drugs in patients with rheumatoid arthritis: A multidatabase cohort study. *Ann. Rheum. Dis.* **2019**, *78*, 456–464. [CrossRef]

23. Kimmig, L.M.; Wu, D.; Gold, M.; Pettit, N.N.; Pitrak, D.; Mueller, J.; Husain, A.N.; Mutlu, E.A.; Mutlu, G.M. IL-6 Inhibition in Critically Ill COVID-19 Patients Is Associated With Increased Secondary Infections. *Front. Med.* **2020**, *7*, 583897. [CrossRef] [PubMed]
24. Shbaklo, N.; Corcione, S.; Vicentini, C.; Giordano, S.; Fiorentino, D.; Bianco, G.; Cattel, F.; Cavallo, R.; Zotti, C.M.; De Rosa, F.G. An Observational Study of MDR Hospital-Acquired Infections and Antibiotic Use during COVID-19 Pandemic: A Call for Antimicrobial Stewardship Programs. *Antibiotics* **2022**, *11*, 695. [CrossRef] [PubMed]
25. Wee, L.E.I.; Conceicao, E.P.; Tan, J.Y.; Magesparan, K.D.; Amin, I.B.M.; Ismail, B.B.S.; Toh, H.X.; Jin, P.; Zhang, J.; Wee, E.G.L.; et al. Unintended consequences of infection prevention and control measures during COVID-19 pandemic. *Am. J. Infect. Control* **2020**, *49*, 469–477. [CrossRef] [PubMed]
26. AlAhdal, A.M.; Alsada, S.A.; Alrashed, H.A.; Al Bazroun, L.I.; Alshoaibi, A. Impact of the COVID-19 Pandemic on Levels of Device-Associated Infections and Hand Hygiene Compliance. *Cureus* **2022**, *14*, e24254. [CrossRef]
27. Basu, M.; Mitra, M.; Ghosh, A.; Pal, R. Prevention of hospital-acquired infections: A construct during Covid-19 pandemic. *J. Fam. Med. Prim. Care* **2021**, *10*, 3348. [CrossRef]
28. Jover-Sáenz, A.; Ramírez-Hidalgo, M.F.; Vidal, M.V.; González, M.G.; Marrón, S.M.C.; Arias, A.E.; Sacrest, M.F.; Castellana-Perelló, D.; Barcenilla-Gaite, F. Antimicrobial stewardship program at a tertiary care academic medical hospital: Clinical, microbiological and economic impact. A 5-year temporary descriptive study. *Infect. Prev. Pr.* **2020**, *2*, 10004. [CrossRef]
29. Davey, P.; A Marwick, C.; Scott, C.L.; Charani, E.; McNeil, K.; Brown, E.; Gould, I.M.; Ramsay, C.R.; Michie, S. Interventions to improve antibiotic prescribing practices for hospital inpatients. *Cochrane Database Syst. Rev.* **2017**, *2017*, CD003543. [CrossRef]
30. Högberg, L.D.; Vlahović-Palčevski, V.; Pereira, C.; Weist, K.; Monnet, D.L. ESAC-Net study group Decrease in community antibiotic consumption during the COVID-19 pandemic, EU/EEA, 2020. *Eurosurveillance* **2021**, *26*, 210102. [CrossRef]
31. Antimicrobial consumption in the EU/EEA (ESAC-Net)—Annual Epidemiological Report for 2020. In: European Centre for Disease Prevention and Control. 2021. Available online: https://www.ecdc.europa.eu/en/publications-data/surveillance-antimicrobial-consumption-europe-2020 (accessed on 25 August 2022).
32. Wunderink, R.G.; Srinivasan, A.; Barie, P.S.; Chastre, J.; Cruz, C.S.D.; Douglas, I.S.; Ecklund, M.; Evans, S.E.; Gerlach, A.T.; Hicks, L.A.; et al. Antibiotic Stewardship in the Intensive Care Unit. An Official American Thoracic Society Workshop Report in Collaboration with the AACN, CHEST, CDC, and SCCM. *Ann. Am. Thorac. Soc.* **2020**, *17*, 531–540. [CrossRef]
33. Kumar, G.; Adams, A.; Hererra, M.; Rojas, E.R.; Singh, V.; Sakhuja, A.; Meersman, M.; Dalton, D.; Kethireddy, S.; Nanchal, R.; et al. Predictors and outcomes of healthcare-associated infections in COVID-19 patients. *Int. J. Infect. Dis.* **2020**, *104*, 287–292. [CrossRef] [PubMed]
34. Gold, J.A.W.; Ahmad, F.B.; A Cisewski, J.; Rossen, L.M.; Montero, A.J.; Benedict, K.; Jackson, B.R.; Toda, M. Increased Deaths From Fungal Infections During the Coronavirus Disease 2019 Pandemic—National Vital Statistics System, United States, January 2020–December 2021. *Clin. Infect. Dis.* **2022**. [CrossRef] [PubMed]
35. Lee, R.A.; Centor, R.M.; Humphrey, L.L.; Jokela, J.A.; Andrews, M.R.; Qaseem, A. Appropriate Use of Short-Course Antibiotics in Common Infections: Best Practice Advice From the American College of Physicians. *Ann. Intern. Med.* **2021**, *174*, 822–827. [CrossRef] [PubMed]

Journal of
Clinical Medicine

MDPI

Article

Bacterial Aspiration Pneumonia in Generalized Convulsive Status Epilepticus: Incidence, Associated Factors and Outcome

Romain Tortuyaux [1,2,*], Frédéric Wallet [3,4], Philippe Derambure [2,5] and Saad Nseir [1,6]

1 Intensive Care Unit, CHU Lille, F-59000 Lille, France
2 Department of Clinical Neurophysiology, CHU Lille, F-59000 Lille, France
3 Laboratoire de Bactériologie-Hygiène, Centre de Biologie Pathologie, CHU Lille, F-59000 Lille, France
4 CNRS, INSERM, Institut Pasteur Lille, U1019-UMR 9017-CIIL, Université de Lille, F-59000 Lille, France
5 CHU Lille, INSERM U1172, Université de Lille, F-59000 Lille, France
6 INSERM U1285, CNRS, UMR 8576-UGSF, Université de Lille, F-59000 Lille, France
* Correspondence: romain.tortuyaux@chu-lille.fr

Abstract: Suspicion of bacterial aspiration pneumonia (BAP) is frequent during generalized convulsive status epilepticus (GCSE). Early identification of BAP is required in order to avoid useless antibiotic therapy. In this retrospective monocentric study, we aimed to determine the incidence of aspiration syndrome and BAP in GCSE requiring mechanical ventilation (MV) and factors associated with the occurrence of BAP. Patients were older than 18 years and had GCSE requiring MV. To distinguish BAP from pneumonitis, tracheal aspirate and quantitative microbiological criterion were used. Out of 226 consecutive patients, 103 patients (46%) had an aspiration syndrome, including 54 (52%) with a BAP. *Staphylococcus aureus* represented 33% of bacterial strains. No relevant baseline characteristics differed, including serum levels of CRP, PCT, and albumin. The median duration of treatment for BAP was 7 days (5–7). Patients with BAP did not have a longer duration of MV ($p = 0.18$) and ICU stay ($p = 0.18$) than those with pneumonitis. At 3 months, 24 patients (44%) with BAP and 10 (27%) with pneumonitis had a poor functional outcome ($p = 0.06$). In conclusion, among patients with GCSE, half of the patients had an aspiration syndrome and one-quarter suffered from BAP. Clinical characteristics and biomarkers were not useful for differentiating BAP from pneumonitis. These results highlight the need for a method to rapidly differentiate BAP from pneumonitis, such as polymerase-chain-reaction-based techniques.

Keywords: status epilepticus; intensive care unit; bacterial aspiration pneumonia; 3-month outcome

Citation: Tortuyaux, R.; Wallet, F.; Derambure, P.; Nseir, S. Bacterial Aspiration Pneumonia in Generalized Convulsive Status Epilepticus: Incidence, Associated Factors and Outcome. *J. Clin. Med.* **2022**, *11*, 6673. https://doi.org/10.3390/jcm11226673

Academic Editors: Tamas Szakmany, Luca Brazzi and Giorgia Montrucchio

Received: 6 September 2022
Accepted: 9 November 2022
Published: 10 November 2022

1. Introduction

Status epilepticus (SE) is broadly defined as a prolonged seizure and remains a common neurological emergency with an overall mortality approaching 20% [1]. Generalized convulsive SE is considered as the worst type of SE and may lead to neurological injury and risk of sequelae [2]. To an early seizure cessation, treatments could be aggressive and contribute to worsening consciousness, such as benzodiazepine or sedatives [3]. In addition, extra-neurological complications are frequent, especially respiratory infection, and may impact the prognosis [4,5]. Aspiration is common in patients with impaired consciousness and is probably more frequent in case of persistent convulsions [6]. Early identification of bacterial aspiration pneumonia (BAP) is needed to avoid useless treatments. In addition, BAP has been associated with acute respiratory distress syndrome and requires an early antibiotic therapy [6]. However, in the absence of a microbiological sample, it is impossible to differentiate BAP from pneumonitis. A previous study in patients with coma requiring MV did not find a relevant difference between patients, highlighting the need for early bacterial identification [7]. To our knowledge, no study has investigated the incidence of BAP and factors associated with the occurrence of BAP in patients with generalized convulsive SE requiring mechanical ventilation (MV).

We hypothesized that the incidence of aspiration syndrome and BAP would be high in a population at risk, as generalized convulsive SE patients are. Therefore, we conducted this retrospective study to determine the incidence of aspiration syndrome and BAP in order to identify factors associated with the occurrence of BAP and to study the impact of aspiration syndrome and BAP on MV duration, intensive care unit (ICU) length of stay, and 3-month outcomes.

2. Materials and Methods

2.1. Patients

From January 2013 to February 2022, we retrospectively screened all patients older than 18 years who were admitted with a diagnosis of status epilepticus to the medical ICU of Lille University Hospital and requiring mechanical ventilation. Patients were screened to confirm the diagnosis of SE—meaning no other possible diagnosis could be considered—and the absence of exclusion criteria.

2.2. Inclusion and Exclusion Criteria

The selected patients had generalized convulsive SE, defined as 5 or more minutes of continuous clinical seizure activity or two seizures without a return to baseline in the interval [2], and had received MV.

Exclusion criteria included post-anoxic SE due to the heterogeneity of their management [8].

According to French law, this database was declared at the institutional data protection board (DEC19-432, DEC20-354), and the study was approved by our local ethics committee (CE SRLF 21-38). This research has therefore been performed in accordance with the ethical standards laid down in the 1964 Declaration of Helsinki and its later amendments. The authors have full access to all data and have the right to publish all data, separate and apart from the guidance of any sponsor.

2.3. Data Collection

For each patient, demographic characteristics and medical history were recorded. Severity at admission was defined using the Simplified Acute Physiology Score II (SAPS II) with exclusion of age studied separately: higher scores indicated greater severity of illness [9]. Clinical characteristics of SE were reported. Refractory status epilepticus was declared if the initial treatment failure included at least one benzodiazepine (i.e., clonazepam) and one intravenous long-duration antiepileptic drug (i.e., fos/phenytoin, levetiracetam, valproic acid, or phenobarbital) prior to intubation [10]. The etiology of SE was defined according to the international league against epilepsy (ILAE) classification: acute (e.g., stroke, intoxication, encephalitis), remote (e.g., poststroke, posttraumatic), progressive (e.g., brain tumor, dementias), and unknown [2]. Psychogenic non-epileptic seizure diagnosis was based on a paroxysmal event without ictal epileptiform EEG changes [11]. Due to a difficult diagnosis at ICU admission and a history of epilepsy frequently associated, these patients were not excluded. We also defined groups of etiology as vascular (acute SE related to ischemic or hemorrhagic stroke, cerebral venous thrombosis, and posterior cerebral encephalopathy), toxic (acute SE related to metabolic disturbance, alcohol, drug intoxication, or withdrawal), and brain tumor (progressive SE related to brain tumor).

Clinical, biological, radiological, and microbiological diagnostic criteria for BAP, as well as clinical outcomes (duration of MV, ICU length of stay, ICU mortality, 3-month mortality, and functional outcome), were collected. Functional outcome was evaluated by modified Rankin Scale (mRS) [12] during a face-to-face visit or by a telephone interview with the patient, the family, or the general practitioner. A poor functional outcome was defined as mRS score > 1 and was different from the pre-SE mRS score.

2.4. Definitions

2.4.1. Aspiration Syndrome

The diagnosis of aspiration syndrome was based on the presence of at least two of the following criteria during the first 2 days after initiation of MV: body temperature of more than 38.5 °C or less than 35.5 °C; leucocyte count greater than 12,000 cells per µL or less than 4000 cells per µL, and purulent tracheal secretions; and the presence of new or progressive infiltrates on the chest X-ray. Chest X-rays were reviewed by at least two attending physicians. In the case of disagreement, a third physician was asked to interpret the chest radiograph. Of note, we collected macroaspiration, defined by history of vomiting before or during intubation, which was not required to define aspiration syndrome.

2.4.2. Bacterial Aspiration Pneumonia, Pneumonitis, and Ventilator-Associated Pneumonia

All aspiration syndromes were classified as [7]

- Bacterial aspiration pneumonia in the case of microbiological confirmation, with the isolation in the endotracheal aspirate of at least 10^5 colony-forming units per mL.
- Pneumonitis, when endotracheal aspirate culture was sterile.

Ventilator-associated pneumonia (VAP) had the same diagnostic criteria as BAP but occurred at least 2 days after starting MV.

2.4.3. Measurements of Serum Levels of C-Reactive Protein (CRP), Procalcitonin (PCT), and Albumin during First 24 h after Admission

CRP was measured with the immunoturbidimetric method and a detection limit of 0.3 mg/L. PCT concentrations were determined using an electrochemiluminescence immunoassay with a detection limit of 0.02 ng/mL. Albumin concentrations were measured with the immunoturbidimetric method. All measurements were performed with Cobas 8000 modular analyzer series (Roche Diagnostics, Rotkreuz, Switzerland).

2.5. Outcomes

The primary outcome was the incidence of bacterial aspiration pneumonia, occurring during the first 2 days after starting invasive MV, among patients admitted to ICU with generalized convulsive SE requiring MV. The secondary outcomes were the incidence of aspiration syndrome in order to identify factors associated with BAP, as well as MV duration, ICU length of stay, functional outcome, and death at 3 months.

2.6. Statistical Analysis

Categorical variables were expressed as numbers and percentages and were compared with the use of ordinal chi-squared or Fisher's exact tests, as appropriate. Continuous variables were expressed as medians (interquartile ranges) and were compared with the use of a *t*-test, Welch's test, or Wilcoxon signed-rank test, as appropriate. A Shapiro–Wilk test was used to distinguish between normal and abnormal distributions.

Logistic multivariable analysis was performed for the occurrence of BAP. To avoid overfitting, only variables with *p*-values under 0.10 in the univariate analysis were considered for inclusion in the final model. Multicollinearity was assessed using variance inflation factor with a cut-off at 4. Clinical relevance of variables was discussed. The fitness was evaluated by Negelkerke's R^2.

All tests were two sided, and the statistical significance was defined by *p*-values under 0.05. Statistical analyses were performed with R statistical software, version 3.6.0 [13].

3. Results

From January 2013 to February 2022, 246 patients were screened for eligibility. Among them, 20 patients with postanoxic SE were excluded. Two hundred and twenty-six patients were admitted to ICU with generalized convulsive SE requiring MV (Figure 1).

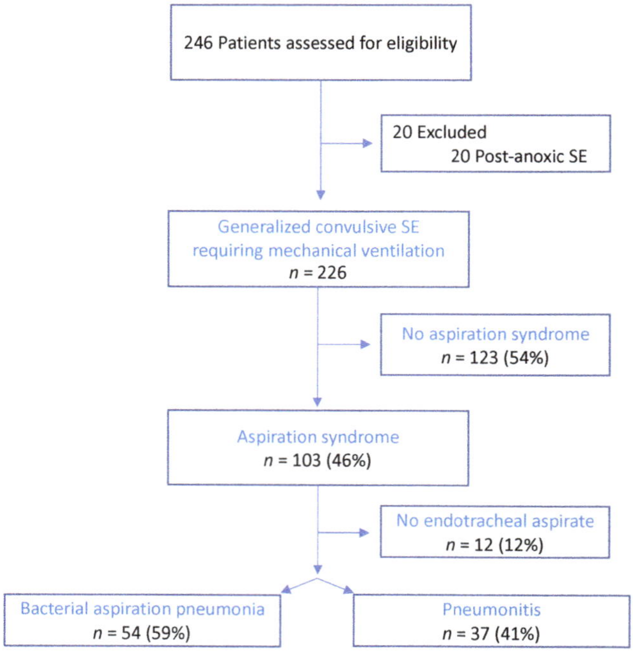

Figure 1. Flowchart. Abbreviations: SE, status epilepticus.

3.1. Patient Characteristics

The median age was 55 years (interquartile range, 43 to 68), and 146 (65%) patients were males. A total of 109 (48%) patients had a history of epilepsy and 40 (18%) of previous SE. Fifty-five (24%) patients were considered as refractory status epilepticus. According to ILAE's etiologic categories, 71 (31%) patients had a SE related to an acute brain injury, 104 (46%) to previous and stable brain lesion (remote symptomatic), 31 (14%) to a progressive brain injury, and 14 (6%) patients had an SE of unknown origin (Table 1).

Table 1. Characteristics and outcomes of patients with and without aspiration syndrome.

Characteristics	Overall Cohort (n = 226)	Aspiration Syndrome (n = 103)	No Aspiration Syndrome (n = 123)	p-Value
Demographics				
Age (years), median (IQR)	55 (43–68)	56 (43–68)	55 (39–67)	0.395
Male sex, n (%)	146 (65)	66 (64)	80 (65)	0.880
mRS score 0–1, n (%)	132 (58)	53 (51)	79 (64)	0.052
SAPS II (without age), median (IQR)	46 (36–54)	50 (34–58)	45 (37–50)	0.113
Medical history, n (%)				
History of epilepsy	109 (48)	50 (49)	59 (48)	0.931
Previous status epilepticus	40 (18)	14 (14)	26 (21)	0.139
Alcohol	83 (37)	43 (42)	40 (33)	0.152
Status epilepticus characteristics, n (%)				
Continuous seizure	72 (32)	32 (31)	40 (33)	0.815
Refractory status epilepticus	55 (24)	22 (21)	33 (27)	0.340
Intubation before ICU admission	128 (57)	56 (54)	72 (59)	0.529
Intubation for respiration failure	130 (58)	57 (55)	73 (59)	0.544
Clinical characteristics at admission				
Core temperature (°C), median (IQR)	36.9 (36.2–37.4)	36.9 (36.2–37.4)	36.8 (36.3–37.4)	0.897
Heart rate (bpm), median (IQR)	97 (80–119)	102 (85–125)	95 (78–112)	**0.011**
Persistent seizures, n (%)	43 (19)	29 (28)	14 (11)	**0.001**
History of macroaspiration, n (%)	23 (10)	12 (12)	11 (9)	0.503
Biological characteristics at admission, median (IQR)				
Leukocyte count (10^9/L)	11.62 (8.88–15.63)	12.12 (9.55–15.67)	11.10 (8.47–15.20)	0.538
Serum CRP level (mg/L)	10 (0–27)	15 (4–36)	6 (0–18)	**0.002**
Serum PCT level (ng/mL)	0.15 (0.00–0.54)	0.18 (0.00–0.91)	0.10 (0.00–0.30)	0.134
Serum albumin level (g/L)	36 (32–40)	35 (31–38)	36 (32–40)	**0.030**
PaO_2/FiO_2 (mmHg)	286 (200–390)	265 (179–335)	313 (223–410)	**<0.001**
Arterial lactate level (mmol/L)	2.1 (1.2–4.0)	2.0 (1.1–3.6)	2.2 (1.3–4.2)	0.569

Table 1. *Cont.*

Characteristics	Overall Cohort (n = 226)	Aspiration Syndrome (n = 103)	No Aspiration Syndrome (n = 123)	p-Value
Etiologic categories, n (%)				
Acute symptomatic	71 (31)	33 (32)	38 (31)	0.853
Remote symptomatic	104 (46)	46 (45)	58 (47)	0.708
Progressive symptomatic	31 (14)	13 (13)	18 (15)	0.661
Unknown	14 (6)	10 (10)	4 (3)	**0.045**
PNES	6 (3)	1 (1)	5 (4)	0.224 *
Main etiologies, n (%)				
Vascular	26 (11)	10 (10)	16 (13)	0.439
Toxic	34 (15)	20 (19)	14 (11)	0.092
Brain tumor	25 (11)	14 (14)	11 (9)	0.267
Outcomes				
Ventilator-associated pneumonia, n (%)	35 (15)	15 (15)	20 (16)	0.725
Mechanical ventilation duration (days), median (IQR)	1.90 (0.88–4.87)	2.71 (1.50–7.10)	1.50 (0.60–3.65)	**0.002**
ICU stay length (days), median (IQR)	4.94 (2.71–9.69)	6.04 (4.23–12.93)	3.90 (2.11–6.92)	**0.011**
ICU mortality, n (%)	11 (5)	7 (7)	4 (3)	0.217
Three-month poor functional outcome, n (%)	78 (35)	38 (38)	40 (33)	0.363
Three-month mortality, n (%)	25 (11)	13 (13)	12 (10)	0.429

Categorical variables were expressed as number (percentage) and compared by a chi-squared test or Fisher's exact test when specified by *. Continuous variables were expressed as a median (inter-quartile range), and a t-test was performed (Welch or Wilcoxon tests, as appropriate). Missing values, overall cohort (aspiration syndrome; no aspiration syndrome): leukocyte count, 3 (0;3); serum CRP level, 20 (6;14); serum PCT level, 50 (19;31); serum albumin level, 21 (9;12); PaO_2/FiO_2, 1 (0;1); lactate arterial level, 3 (1;2); 3-month outcomes, 4 (4;0). Abbreviations: mRS, modified Rankin scale; SAPS II, simplified acute physiology score; ICU, intensive care unit; CRP, C-reactive protein; PCT, procalcitonin; PNES, psychogenic non-epileptic seizure.

3.2. Comparison of Patients with and without Aspiration Syndrome

One hundred and three patients (46%) met the criteria for aspiration syndrome. Of note, considering the overall cohort, these criteria were frequently found during the first 48 h of MV: 147 (66%) had abnormal body temperature, 160 (72%) had purulent tracheal aspirates, and 171 (77%) had leukocytosis.

At admission, patients with aspiration syndrome had more frequently persistent seizures ($p = 0.001$). Body temperature was similar ($p = 0.90$) and heart rate was higher in patients with aspiration syndrome ($p = 0.01$). No other baseline characteristics differed, especially SE characteristics and etiology. Interestingly, macroaspiration ($p = 0.50$) and timing ($p = 0.53$) or reason ($p = 0.54$) for intubation were not associated with aspiration syndrome (Table 1).

Regarding laboratory results, patients with aspiration syndrome had a lower $Pa0_2/Fi0_2$ ratio ($p < 0.001$), a higher serum level of CRP ($p < 0.01$), and a lower serum level of albumin ($p = 0.03$). No difference was found for serum blood level of PCT ($p = 0.13$) and leukocyte count ($p = 0.54$) (Table 1).

Aspiration syndrome was associated with a longer MV duration ($p < 0.01$) and ICU length of stay ($p = 0.01$). Three-month mortality ($p = 0.43$) and poor functional outcome ($p = 0.36$) did not differ between groups (Table 1).

3.3. Comparison of Patients with BAP versus Pneumonitis

Among patients with aspiration syndrome, 12 (5%) did not have endotracheal aspirate and could not be classified as BAP or pneumonitis. These patients were excluded for analysis concerning BAP and pneumonitis (Figure 1). Fifty-four patients (59%) had a BAP, whereas others were considered as pneumonitis. Considering the overall cohort, 24% of patients with GCSE presented a BAP.

Patients with BAP, in comparison with pneumonitis, were less likely alcoholic ($p = 0.02$) and had a higher SAPS II at admission ($p = 0.03$). No other baseline characteristics differed, especially SE characteristics and etiology (Table 2).

Table 2. Comparison of patients' characteristics according to the diagnosis of BAP or pneumonitis.

Characteristics	BAP ($n = 54$)	Pneumonitis ($n = 37$)	p-Value
Demographics			
Age (years), median (IQR)	55 (42–67)	65 (48–71)	0.126
Male sex, n (%)	37 (69)	25 (68)	0.924
mRS score 0–1, n (%)	26 (48)	21 (57)	0.420
SAPS II (without age), median (IQR)	51 (38–58)	44 (28–58)	**0.035**
Medical history, n (%)			
History of epilepsy	25 (46)	18 (49)	0.825
Previous status epilepticus	4 (7)	9 (24)	**0.023**
Alcohol	17 (31)	21 (57)	**0.016**
Use of proton pump inhibitor	19 (35)	13 (35)	0.996
Status epilepticus characteristics, n (%)			
Continuous seizure	17 (31)	11 (30)	0.859
Refractory status epilepticus	11 (20)	9 (24)	0.655
Intubation before ICU admission	29 (54)	21 (57)	0.774
Intubation for respiration failure	34 (63)	17 (46)	0.108
Clinical characteristics at admission			
Core temperature (°C), median (IQR)	36.8 (36.1–37.1)	37.0 (36.3–37.8)	0.095
Heart rate (bpm), median (IQR)	96 (81–120)	111 (90–124)	0.191
Persistent seizures, n (%)	15 (28)	10 (27)	0.937
History of macroaspiration, n (%)	4 (7)	6 (16)	0.306 *

Table 2. *Cont.*

Characteristics	BAP (n = 54)	Pneumonitis (n = 37)	p-Value
Biological characteristics at admission, median (IQR)			
Leukocyte count (10^9/L)	12.28 (9.58–15.31)	11.88 (9.53–15.68)	0.792
Serum CRP level (mg/L)	12 (2–36)	13 (0–31)	0.777
Serum PCT level (ng/mL)	0.17 (0.00–0.63)	0.14 (0.00–0.53)	0.869
Serum albumin level (g/L)	35 (32–39)	35 (31–37)	0.411
PaO_2/FiO_2 (mmHg)	281 (185–391)	263 (192–314)	0.344
Arterial lactate level (mmol/L)	1.85 (1.00–3.17)	2.40 (1.42–4.92)	0.306
Etiologic categories, n (%)			
Acute symptomatic	15 (28)	13 (35)	0.455
Remote symptomatic	24 (44)	16 (43)	0.910
Progressive symptomatic	8 (15)	4 (11)	0.755 *
Unknown	6 (11)	4 (11)	0.964 *
Main etiologies, n (%)			
Vascular	5 (9)	2 (5)	0.696 *
Toxic	9 (17)	9 (24)	0.368
Brain tumor	8 (15)	5 (14)	0.862

Categorical variables were expressed as number (percentage) and compared by a chi-squared test or Fisher's exact test when specified by *. Continuous variables were expressed as median (inter-quartile range), and a t-test was performed (Welch or Wilcoxon tests, as appropriate). Missing values (BAP; pneumonitis): CRP, 6 (5;1); PCT, 19 (12;7); albumin, 7 (3;4); lactate arterial, 1 (0;1). Abbreviations: BAP, bacterial aspiration pneumonia; mRS, modified Rankin scale; SAPS II, simplified acute physiology score; ICU, intensive care unit; CRP, C-reactive protein; PCT, procalcitonin.

We found no difference concerning serum levels of CRP (p = 0.78), PCT (p = 0.87), and albumin (p = 0.41) between patients with BAP and pneumonitis. The severity of hypoxia estimated by the $Pa0_2/Fi0_2$ ratio and arterial lactate level did not differ between groups (respectively, p = 0.34 and p = 0.31) (Table 2).

We did not perform a multivariable analysis due to the absence of clinical relevance.

3.4. Etiology of Bacterial Aspiration Pneumonia

Of the 54 patients with BAP, 71 different bacterial strains were identified. They are presented in Table 3 with their antimicrobial susceptibility. Fifteen (28%) patients had a polymicrobial BAP. The most represented bacteria were *Staphylococcus aureus* (18; 33%), *Haemophilus influenzae* (13; 24%), *Streptococcus pneumoniae* (10; 19%) and *Klebsiella pneumoniae* (9; 17%).

Table 3. Bacterial strains identified by endotracheal aspirate in patients with bacterial aspiration pneumonia.

Type of Bacteria	Bacteria	Number of Isolates, n (%)	Resistance
Gram+ (30 bacteria isolated from 29 patients, 54 %)			
***Staphylococcus* spp.**	*Staphylococcus aureus*	18 (33)	Methicillin-sensitive: 16 (penicillin-resistant: 8, tested in 10 isolates) Methicillin-resistant: 2 *
***Streptococcus* spp.**	*Streptococcus pneumoniae*	10 (19)	Wild-type: 6 Decreased susceptibility to penicillin: 4
	Streptococcus agalactiae	2 (4)	Wild-type: 2

Table 3. *Cont.*

Type of Bacteria	Bacteria	Number of Isolates, *n* (%)	Resistance
	Gram− (41 bacteria isolated from 36 patients, 67 %)		
Group 1, 2, and 5 enterobacterales	*Klebsiella pneumoniae*	9 (17)	Wild-type: 6 β-Lactamase: 1 * ESBL: 2 *
	Escherichia coli	7 (13)	Wild-type: 3 Low-production of β-lactamase: 1 Hyperproduction of β-lactamase: 3 *
	Klebsiella oxytoca	1 (2)	Wild-type: 1
	Proteus vulgaris	1 (2)	Wild-type: 1
Group 3 enterobacterales	*Enterobacter cloacae*	2 (4)	Wild-type: 1 * ESBL: 1 *
	Hafnia alvei	1 (2)	Wild-type: 1 *
Non-fermenting bacilli	*Pseudomonas aeruginosa*	2 (4)	Wild-type: 2 *
	Acinetobacter baumannii	1 (2)	Wild-type: 1 *
Other bacteria	*Haemophilus influenzae*	13 (24)	Wild-type: 12 β-Lactamase: 1
	Moraxella catarrhalis	2 (4)	β-Lactamase: 1 Wild-type: 1
	Lelliottia amnigena	1 (2)	ACA-resistant: 1 *
	Pasteurella multocida	1 (2)	Wild-type: 1

Of the 54 patients with BAP, 71 different bacterial strains were identified. Antimicrobial susceptibility was defined, and * corresponds to ACA-resistant bacteria. Abbreviations: ESBL, extended spectrum beta-lactamase; ACA, amoxicillin-clavulanic acid.

3.5. Antibiotic Therapy

A total of 158 patients (70%) were treated by antibiotic therapy: 138 (87%) for suspicion of BAP and 20 (13%) for documented or suspected infection other than BAP.

Among patients with suspicion of BAP, 45 patients (33%) did not have an aspiration syndrome and 120 (87%) were treated by ACA.

Among the 54 patients with BAP, 13 (24%) patients presented at least one bacterium with no ACA-susceptibility. These patients more frequently had a colonization with ESBL-producing bacteria ($p = 0.01$) and received more antibiotics during the 3 months before ICU admission ($p < 0.01$) (Supplementary Materials Table S1). Among them, initial antibiotic therapy was inappropriate in 11 patients (85%). None presented an acute respiratory syndrome distress, or a septic shock or death related to respiratory infection.

The median duration of treatment for BAP was 7 days (5–7). In comparison with BAP, patients with pneumonitis did not have a shorter duration of antibiotic therapy ($p = 0.46$).

3.6. Outcomes of BAP Versus Pneumonitis

Patients with BAP, as compared with those with pneumonitis, did not have a longer duration of MV ($p = 0.18$) and ICU stay ($p = 0.18$). Three-month mortality was 17% versus 8%, respectively, in patients with BAP and pneumonitis ($p = 0.20$). Twenty-four patients (44%) in the BAP group versus ten (27%) in pneumonitis group had a 3-month poor functional outcome ($p = 0.06$) (Table 4).

Table 4. Comparison of patients' outcomes according to the diagnosis of BAP or pneumonitis.

Characteristics	BAP (n = 54)	Pneumonitis (n = 37)	p-Value
Ventilator-associated pneumonia, n (%)	10 (19)	4 (11)	0.317
Mechanical ventilation duration (days), median (IQR)	3.39 (1.71–8.35)	2.37 (0.83–6.88)	0.179
ICU stay length (days), median (IQR)	6.83 (4.38–13.25)	6.46 (3.58–12.50)	0.180
ICU mortality, n (%)	6 (11)	1 (3)	0.234 *
Three-month poor functional outcome, n (%)	24 (44)	10 (27)	0.057
Three-month mortality, n (%)	9 (17)	3 (8)	0.198

Categorical variables were expressed as number (percentage) and compared by a chi-squared test or Fisher's exact test when specified by *. Continuous variables were expressed as median (inter-quartile range), and a t-test was performed (Welch or Wilcoxon tests, as appropriate). Missing values (BAP; pneumonitis): 3-month outcomes, 3 (3;0). Abbreviations: BAP, bacterial aspiration pneumonia; ICU, intensive care unit.

4. Discussion

In the present study, we found the following: (1) Half the patients with generalized convulsive SE requiring mechanical ventilation had an aspiration syndrome and one-quarter suffered from BAP. (2) No clinical and laboratory characteristics allowed for the separation of BAP from pneumonitis. In particular, biomarkers related to inflammatory response such as serum CRP, PCT, and albumin were not associated with BAP and rather were modified by aspiration syndrome, including pneumonitis. (3) Up to one-quarter of bacteria isolated from tracheal samples was not sensitive to ACA, with no clinical consequence (i.e., septic shock, acute respiratory distress syndrome). (4) Finally, we did not find that BAP was associated with a poor functional outcome and death at 3 months compared to pneumonitis.

Aspiration syndrome is a frequent condition occurring in cases of impairment of consciousness [14]. In comparison with patients requiring MV for coma (epilepsy was the etiology of coma in 14%), we found a higher frequency of aspiration syndrome and BAP [7]. This result could be related to a higher risk of aspiration during SE. Indeed, in our study, persistent convulsions at admission were associated with aspiration syndrome. In another study of patients requiring MV for coma (13% had a convulsive SE), the authors found a higher frequency of aspiration syndrome (81 patients, 79%) and more BAP (45 patients, 44%) than in our cohort [15].

As previously described, aspiration syndrome was responsible for a longer duration of MV and ICU stay, without impact on ICU mortality [7].

Differentiation BAP from pneumonitis is the keystone of antibiotic management in order to avoid useless prescriptions and the emergence of resistant bacteria. In line with a previous study, we found no relevant difference between BAP and pneumonitis, including previous use of a proton pump inhibitor [7,16]. Serum levels of acute-phase proteins of inflammation were not modified by BAP. PCT increases under various inflammatory conditions, especially in the case of bacterial infections [17,18]. Some studies tried to use PCT to distinguish pneumonitis from BAP with no significant difference [7,19]. Only one study found that serum levels of CRP and PCT increased in cases of BAP with a poor diagnostic value [15]. However, they compared BAP versus no BAP (including pneumonitis and absence of aspiration syndrome), and the results could be biased by the presence of patients without aspiration syndrome who do not have increased serum levels of CRP and PCT [15]. Interestingly, early elevation of PCT is rather associated with poor neurological outcome in acute brain injury, such as SE [20,21], post-cardiac arrest syndrome [22], and stroke [23]. Currently, only microbiological culture of the tracheal sample differentiates these two entities with a result obtained in 2–3 days [24]. One elegant method to rapidly differentiate pneumonitis from BAP is to use polymerase chain reaction (PCR)-based techniques [25,26]. The results could be obtained in a few hours, reducing antimicrobial consumption in the ICU and breaking the vicious circle of multidrug-resistant bacteria emergence [27]. Furthermore, in the case of SE, some experimental and clinical data suggest that antibiotic therapy could increase the risk of symptomatic seizures in combination with renal dysfunction, brain lesion, and epilepsy [28].

Microbiology of BAP with a predominance of *Staphylococcus aureus*, *Haemophilus influenzae*, and *Streptococcus pneumoniae* is in line with a previous study [29].

Infections in SE are already known as factors associated with poor outcome [5]. The impact on MV duration and ICU stay is uncertain, in contrast to aspiration syndrome, but could be increased in BAP [7,15]. Further, previous studies reported the absence of significant relationship between BAP and ICU mortality [7,15]. However, our study follow-up at 3 months highlighted a possible higher mortality and morbidity in BAP versus pneumonitis. A large prospective study is needed to confirm these results.

Antibiotic therapy was frequently initiated for suspicion of BAP. However, one-third of patients did not have aspiration syndrome. Two reasons could explain this early antibiotic treatment: the presence of macroaspiration [30] and the elevation of inflammatory biomarkers such as serum levels of CRP and PCT. We found that macroaspiration, defined by history of vomiting before or during intubation, was not predictive of aspiration syndrome; and modifications of acute-phase proteins of inflammation, such as CRP and PCT were associated with aspiration syndrome rather than BAP.

One-quarter of patients with BAP had at least one bacterium that was non-susceptible to ACA. ACA, as alternative to ceftriaxone, is recommended for treatment of respiratory infection occurring during the first 5 days after admission [31]. Antibiotics before ICU admission and colonization with ESBL-producing bacterium are well known factors associated with ACA resistance [31]. In another study of early onset VAP (2–5 days after mechanical ventilation starting, corresponding to ICU admission) in a French neuro-ICU, the authors found 36% of patients with at least one bacterium resistant to ACA, mainly in patients with antibiotics before admission [32]. These data are in line with previous studies [31]. It seems important to determine new specific factors associated with ACA resistance and to develop a PCR-based method to rapidly identify antimicrobial resistance.

The median duration of antibiotic therapy for suspicion of BAP was 7 days, in line with the actual recommendation [33]. However, in the case of pneumonitis, we did not show a shorter duration, probably due to the delay in obtaining the result of microbiological culture and the fear of false-negative results [30]. In one study of patients with coma requiring MV, discontinuation of antibiotic therapy when no microorganism was found did not increase morbidity or mortality and tended to decrease the time with antibiotics during first 8 days [7]. The excellent predictive value of PCR-based methods would be interesting to use early on to differentiate pneumonitis from BAP, in order to avoid antibiotic treatment or to allow early withdrawal in patients with negative results and so decrease antibiotic consumption. This strategy is being studied in an ongoing randomized controlled trial (NCT03763799).

Our study has some strengths. Patients were similar in their clinical presentation with only GCSE. Post-anoxic SE was excluded due to the heterogeneity of their management [8]. The monocentric design contributed to a homogeneous management, especially in SE treatment and BAP diagnosis. Baseline characteristics and the main results were in line with previous studies [7,15]. Infection was considered only when confirmed by culture.

Our study also has some limitations. Monocentric design contributes to the small size of the cohort and results should be applied only for generalized convulsive SE. However, our main results are similar to those of a study including different causes of coma [7]. The long duration of data collection could impact the results. However, the methodology to determine infection did not change during the study. The primary outcome was the incidence of bacterial aspiration pneumonia, and a potential modification of bacterial ecology could not affect this variable. We did not have a control group to compare incidence of BAP between patients with SE and patients with impaired consciousness not due to SE. No anaerobic microorganisms were identified by microbiological cultures. They may play a role in BAP; however, they are often mixed with aerobic bacteria [29].

5. Conclusions

In conclusion, among patients with generalized convulsive SE requiring MV, half had criteria for aspiration syndrome and one-quarter of patients had a BAP. Clinical characteristics and biomarkers, such as serum CRP, PCT, and albumin levels measured during the first 24 h, were not useful to differentiate BAP from pneumonitis. Up to one-quarter of bacteria isolated from tracheal samples were not sensitive to ACA, with no clinical consequences despite inappropriate antibiotic therapy. BAP tended to be associated with poor functional outcome and death at 3 months. Our results highlight the need for a method to rapidly differentiate pneumonitis from BAP, such as PCR-based techniques.

Supplementary Materials: The following supporting information can be downloaded at https://www.mdpi.com/article/10.3390/jcm11226673/s1, Table S1: Comparison of patients with BAP according to amoxicillin/clavulanic acid susceptibility among causative pathogens.

Author Contributions: Conceptualization, R.T. and S.N.; methodology, R.T.; validation, R.T., F.W. and S.N.; formal analysis, R.T. and S.N.; data curation, R.T., F.W. and P.D.; writing—original draft preparation, R.T.; writing—review and editing, R.T., F.W., P.D. and S.N. All authors have read and agreed to the published version of the manuscript.

Funding: This research received no external funding.

Institutional Review Board Statement: The study was conducted in accordance with the Declaration of Helsinki and approved by the Ethics Committee of SRLF (French Society of Intensive Care) (protocol code CE SRLF 21-38 and date of approval: 3 September 2022).

Informed Consent Statement: Informed consent was obtained from all subjects involved in the study.

Data Availability Statement: The data presented in this study are available on request from the corresponding author. The data are not publicly available due to privacy reasons.

Conflicts of Interest: S.N. received payment for lectures from MSD, Pfizer, Gilead, Biomérieux, Bio Rad, and Fischer and Paykel. R.T., F.W. and P.D. declare no conflict of interest.

References

1. Betjemann, J.P.; Lowenstein, D.H. Status Epilepticus in Adults. *Lancet Neurol.* **2015**, *14*, 615–624. [CrossRef]
2. Trinka, E.; Cock, H. A Definition and Classification of Status Epilepticus—Report of the ILAE Task Force on Classification of Status Epilepticus. *Epilepsia* **2015**, *56*, 1515–1523. [CrossRef] [PubMed]
3. Kapur, J.; Elm, J. Randomized Trial of Three Anticonvulsant Medications for Status Epilepticus. *N. Engl. J. Med.* **2019**, *381*, 2103–2113. [CrossRef] [PubMed]
4. Sutter, R.; Dittrich, T. Acute Systemic Complications of Convulsive Status Epilepticus-A Systematic Review. *Crit. Care Med.* **2018**, *46*, 138–145. [CrossRef]
5. Semmlack, S.; Tschudin-Sutter, S. Independent Impact of Infections on the Course and Outcome of Status Epilepticus: A 10-Year Cohort Study. *J. Neurol.* **2016**, *263*, 1303–1313. [CrossRef]
6. DiBardino, D.M.; Wunderink, R.G. Aspiration Pneumonia: A Review of Modern Trends. *J. Crit. Care* **2015**, *30*, 40–48. [CrossRef]
7. Lascarrou, J.B.; Lissonde, F. Antibiotic Therapy in Comatose Mechanically Ventilated Patients Following Aspiration: Differentiating Pneumonia from Pneumonitis. *Crit. Care Med.* **2017**, *45*, 1268–1275. [CrossRef]
8. Ruijter, B.J.; Keijzer, H.M. Treating Rhythmic and Periodic EEG Patterns in Comatose Survivors of Cardiac Arrest. *N. Engl. J. Med.* **2022**, *386*, 724–734. [CrossRef]
9. Le Gall, J.-R.; Lemeshow, S. A New Simplified Acute Physiology Score (SAPS II) Based on a European/North American Multicenter Study. *JAMA* **1993**, *270*, 2957. [CrossRef]
10. Rossetti, A.O.; Lowenstein, D.H. Management of Refractory Status Epilepticus in Adults: Still More Questions than Answers. *Lancet Neurol.* **2011**, *10*, 922–930. [CrossRef]
11. Mezouar, N.; Demeret, S. Psychogenic Non-Epileptic Seizure-Status in Patients Admitted to the Intensive Care Unit. *Eur. J. Neurol.* **2021**, *28*, 2775–2779. [CrossRef] [PubMed]
12. Van Swieten, J.C.; Koudstaal, P.J. Interobserver Agreement for the Assessment of Handicap in Stroke Patients. *Stroke* **1988**, *19*, 604–607. [CrossRef] [PubMed]
13. *R Core Team R: A Language and Environment for Statistical Computing*; R Foundation for Statistical Computing: Vienna, Austria, 2019.
14. Neill, S.; Dean, N. Aspiration Pneumonia and Pneumonitis: A Spectrum of Infectious/Noninfectious Diseases Affecting the Lung. *Curr. Opin. Infect. Dis.* **2019**, *32*, 152–157. [CrossRef]

15. Legriel, S.; Grigoresco, B. Diagnostic Accuracy of Procalcitonin for Early Aspiration Pneumonia in Critically Ill Patients with Coma: A Prospective Study. *Neurocrit. Care* **2019**, *30*, 440–448. [CrossRef] [PubMed]
16. Herzig, S.J.; Howell, M.D. Acid-Suppressive Medication Use and the Risk for Hospital-Acquired Pneumonia. *JAMA* **2009**, *301*, 2120–2128. [CrossRef]
17. Becker, K.L.; Snider, R. Procalcitonin in Sepsis and Systemic Inflammation: A Harmful Biomarker and a Therapeutic Target. *Br. J. Pharmacol.* **2010**, *159*, 253–264. [CrossRef] [PubMed]
18. De Kruif, M.D.; Limper, M. Additional Value of Procalcitonin for Diagnosis of Infection in Patients with Fever at the Emergency Department. *Crit. Care Med.* **2010**, *38*, 457–463. [CrossRef]
19. El-Solh, A.A.; Vora, H. Diagnostic Use of Serum Procalcitonin Levels in Pulmonary Aspiration Syndromes. *Crit. Care Med.* **2011**, *39*, 1251–1256. [CrossRef]
20. Sutter, R.; Valença, M. Procalcitonin and Mortality in Status Epilepticus: An Observational Cohort Study. *Crit. Care* **2015**, *19*, 361. [CrossRef]
21. Sutter, R.; Grize, L. Acute-Phase Proteins and Mortality in Status Epilepticus: A 5-Year Observational Cohort Study. *Crit. Care Med.* **2013**, *41*, 1526–1533. [CrossRef]
22. Engel, H.; ben Hamouda, N. Serum Procalcitonin as a Marker of Post-Cardiac Arrest Syndrome and Long-Term Neurological Recovery, but Not of Early-Onset Infections, in Comatose Post-Anoxic Patients Treated with Therapeutic Hypothermia. *Resuscitation* **2013**, *84*, 776–781. [CrossRef] [PubMed]
23. Deng, W.-J.; Shen, R.-L. Relationship between Procalcitonin Serum Levels and Functional Outcome in Stroke Patients. *Cell Mol. Neurobiol.* **2015**, *35*, 355–361. [CrossRef] [PubMed]
24. Bretonnière, C.; Leone, M. Strategies to Reduce Curative Antibiotic Therapy in Intensive Care Units (Adult and Paediatric). *Intensive Care Med.* **2015**, *41*, 1181–1196. [CrossRef] [PubMed]
25. Clavel, M.; Barraud, O. Molecular Quantification of Bacteria from Respiratory Samples in Patients with Suspected Ventilator-Associated Pneumonia. *Clin. Microbiol. Infect.* **2016**, *22*, 812.e1–812.e7. [CrossRef]
26. Tortuyaux, R.; Voisin, B. Could Polymerase Chain Reaction-Based Methods Differentiate Pneumonitis from Bacterial Aspiration Pneumonia? *Crit. Care Med.* **2018**, *46*, e96–e97. [CrossRef]
27. Dragan, V.; Wei, Y. Prophylactic Antimicrobial Therapy for Acute Aspiration Pneumonitis. *Clin. Infect. Dis.* **2018**, *67*, 513–518. [CrossRef]
28. Sutter, R.; Rüegg, S. Seizures as Adverse Events of Antibiotic Drugs: A Systematic Review. *Neurology* **2015**, *85*, 1332–1341. [CrossRef]
29. Lauterbach, E.; Voss, F. Bacteriology of Aspiration Pneumonia in Patients with Acute Coma. *Intern. Emerg. Med.* **2014**, *9*, 879–885. [CrossRef]
30. Rebuck, J.A.; Rasmussen, J.R. Clinical Aspiration-Related Practice Patterns in the Intensive Care Unit: A Physician Survey. *Crit. Care Med.* **2001**, *29*, 2239–2244. [CrossRef]
31. Torres, A.; Niederman, M.S. International ERS/ESICM/ESCMID/ALAT Guidelines for the Management of Hospital-Acquired Pneumonia and Ventilator-Associated Pneumonia. *Eur. Respir. J.* **2017**, *50*, 1700582. [CrossRef]
32. Premachandra, A.; Mazeraud, A. Is Amoxicillin/Clavulanic Acid the Best Option to Treat Early-Onset Ventilator-Acquired Pneumonia in Brain-Injured Patients. *J. Glob Antimicrob. Resist.* **2021**, *27*, 247–249. [CrossRef] [PubMed]
33. Mandell, L.A.; Niederman, M.S. Aspiration Pneumonia. *N. Engl. J. Med.* **2019**, *380*, 651–663. [CrossRef] [PubMed]

Journal of
Clinical Medicine

MDPI

Article

Dose Optimization of Meropenem in Patients on Veno-Arterial Extracorporeal Membrane Oxygenation in Critically Ill Cardiac Patients: Pharmacokinetic/Pharmacodynamic Modeling

Soyoung Kang [1,2], Seungwon Yang [2,3,4], Jongsung Hahn [2,5], June Young Jang [1], Kyoung Lok Min [1], Jin Wi [6,7,*,†] and Min Jung Chang [1,2,8,*,†]

1 Department of Pharmaceutical Medicine and Regulatory Science, Yonsei University, Incheon 21983, Korea
2 Department of Pharmacy and Yonsei Institute of Pharmaceutical Sciences, Yonsei University, Incheon 21983, Korea
3 Department of Pharmacy, College of Pharmacy, Kyung Hee University, Seoul 02447, Korea
4 Department of Regulatory Science, College of Pharmacy, Graduate School, Kyung Hee University, Seoul 02447, Korea
5 School of Pharmacy, Jeonbuk National University, Jeonju 54896, Korea
6 Division of Cardiology, Department of Internal Medicine, Gachon University Gil Medical Center, Incheon 21565, Korea
7 Division of Cardiology, Department of Internal Medicine, Yonsei University College of Medicine, Seoul 03722, Korea
8 Graduate Program of Industrial Pharmaceutical Science, Yonsei University, Incheon 21983, Korea
* Correspondence: caesar@gilhospital.com or caesar@yuhs.ac (J.W.); mjchang@yonsei.ac.kr (M.J.C.); Tel.: +82-32-460-3663 (J.W); +82-32-749-4517 (M.J.C.); Fax: +82-32-749-4105 (M.J.C.)
† These authors contributed equally to this work.

Citation: Kang, S.; Yang, S.; Hahn, J.; Jang, J.Y.; Min, K.L.; Wi, J.; Chang, M.J. Dose Optimization of Meropenem in Patients on Veno-Arterial Extracorporeal Membrane Oxygenation in Critically Ill Cardiac Patients: Pharmacokinetic/Pharmacodynamic Modeling. *J. Clin. Med.* **2022**, *11*, 6621. https://doi.org/10.3390/jcm11226621

Academic Editors: Luca Brazzi and Giorgia Montrucchio

Received: 10 October 2022
Accepted: 2 November 2022
Published: 8 November 2022

Publisher's Note: MDPI stays neutral with regard to jurisdictional claims in published maps and institutional affiliations.

Abstract: Background: Our objective was to determine an optimal dosage regimen of meropenem in patients receiving veno-arterial extracorporeal membrane oxygenation (V-A ECMO) by developing a pharmacokinetic/pharmacodynamic (PK/PD) model. Methods: This was a prospective cohort study. Blood samples were collected during ECMO (ECMO-ON) and after ECMO (ECMO-OFF). The population pharmacokinetic model was developed using nonlinear mixed-effects modeling. A Monte Carlo simulation was used (n = 10,000) to assess the probability of target attainment. Results: Thirteen adult patients on ECMO receiving meropenem were included. Meropenem pharmacokinetics was best fitted by a two-compartment model. The final pharmacokinetic model was: CL (L/h) = 3.79×0.44^{CRRT}, central volume of distribution (L) = 2.4, peripheral volume of distribution (L) = 8.56, and intercompartmental clearance (L/h) = 21.3. According to the simulation results, if more aggressive treatment is needed (100% $fT > MIC$ target), dose increment or extended infusion is recommended. Conclusions: We established a population pharmacokinetic model for meropenem in patients receiving V-A ECMO and revealed that it is not necessary to adjust the dosage depending on V-A ECMO. Instead, more aggressive treatment is needed than that of standard treatment, and higher dosage is required without continuous renal replacement therapy (CRRT). Also, extended infusion could lead to better target attainment, and we could provide updated nomograms of the meropenem dosage regimen.

Keywords: meropenem; extracorporeal membrane oxygenation; ECMO; dosage optimization; population pharmacokinetics

1. Introduction

Veno-arterial extracorporeal membrane oxygenation (V-A ECMO) provides mechanical circulatory support for patients with cardiopulmonary failure [1]. There have been exponential increases in ECMO use and survival rates since 2009 [2]. However, infection is still a common complication during ECMO because it requires the use of percutaneously inserted devices with large-diameter catheters, and critically ill patients themselves are generally vulnerable to infection [2,3]. One observation study reported that 62.8% had a bloodstream infection within 2 weeks of V-A ECMO, and both gram-positive and gram-negative bacteremia commonly occurred [4]. Biaazrro et al. also reported that the prevalence of infection in adult patients with ECMO was 21%, which was higher than that of children (16%) and neonates (8%). Also, V-A ECMO has higher risk of infectious complications than V-V ECMO [5]. Therefore, successful prevention and treatment of infection by broad-spectrum antibiotics is necessary in patients receiving V-A ECMO is [2,6].

It is well known that V-A ECMO affects the pharmacokinetics (PK) of several drugs [7], altering their volume of distribution (Vd) and clearance (CL) because of inherent physiological changes associated with ECMO and critical illness [8–10]. Non-pulsatile blood flow from V-A ECMO reduces glomerular filtration rate, and consequently reduces the CL of drugs [11]. Patients with profound cardiogenic shock during V-A ECMO commonly need more aggressive volume support for hemodynamic stabilization [12], which widely alters the effect of ECMO treatment on PK parameters. In addition, PK changes in patients receiving ECMO are dependent on the physicochemical properties of the drugs [13]. Therefore, exact predictions of PK changes in V-A ECMO are difficult [14].

One of the commonly used broad-spectrum antibiotics, piperacillin-tazobactam, was studied, and ECMO and CRRT increased, with Vd and the use of ECMO reduced CL [15]. The other study reported that use of ECMO increased both CL and Vd of cefpirome, another broad-spectrum antibiotic. However, studies on the impact of ECMO on meropenem PK showed conflicting results [16,17]. Shekar et al. reported that the CL was reduced during ECMO, but Gijsen et al. said that the use of ECMO did not influence the PKs of meropenem.

Thus, the present study aims to describe the PK profiles of meropenem by comparing patients receiving V-A ECMO with patients after stopping ECMO treatment. In addition, optimal dosage regimens were determined according to individual characteristics by simulating various dosing scenarios in patients on both V-A ECMO and continuous renal replacement therapy (CRRT).

2. Methods

This prospective cohort study was conducted from May 2016 to January 2019 in the cardiac intensive care unit of Severance Hospital in Seoul, Korea. Adult patients (≥18 years) receiving V-A ECMO and concomitantly receiving meropenem were included in this study. Patients who were allergic to carbapenem or pregnant were excluded. Patients with normal kidney function received 1 g meropenem q8h as an intravenous injection over 20 min as per protocol. Patients with an estimated glomerular filtration rate (eGFR) of less than 30 mL/min/1.73 m^2, as calculated by the Modification of Diet in Renal Disease (MDRD) study equation, or patients on CRRT, received 1 g meropenem q12h.

The ECMO system consisted of a centrifugal blood pump with a controller (Capiox® SP-101, Terumo Inc., Tokyo, Japan), a conduit tube (Capiox® EBS with X coating, Terumo Inc., Tokyo, Japan), and an air-oxygen mixer (Sechrist® Industries, Inc., Anaheim, CA, USA). It was connected percutaneously between the femoral vein and peripheral cannulation of the femoral artery. If needed, continuous venovenous hemodiafiltration (CV-VHDF) (Prismaflex®; Gambro Inc., Meyzieu, France) with a Prismaflex® ST100 filter was utilized for CRRT. The ECMO and CRRT settings were recorded.

Data associated with demographics, renal and hepatic functions, blood chemistry, vital signs, blood cell counts, and details of ECMO and CRRT were collected. As allowed by the clinical situation, blood samples were collected during ECMO (ECMO-ON group) through the existing radial arterial line at the following times: pre-dose (0 min); 0.5, 1, 3, and 6 h after meropenem administration; and immediately before the next dose, according to administration frequency (8 h or 12 h). If the patients were administered meropenem after them weaning off of ECMO (ECMO-OFF group), blood samples were collected at the aforementioned times. The actual sampling time was recorded. The blood samples were collected in EDTA-coated tubes and immediately centrifuged (1500× *g* at 4 °C for 10 min). The plasma samples were stored at −80 °C until analysis.

Meropenem concentrations were measured using liquid chromatography-mass spectrometry (LC-MS, Ultimate 3000 RS-Q-Exactive Orbitrap Plus; Thermo Fisher Scientific, Waltham, MA, USA) in the Yonsei Center for Research Facilities. The plasma samples were deproteinized using acetonitrile with sulfamethoxine as an internal standard. The mixture was vortexed for 10 s, and then centrifuged (10 min at 10,000× *g*), and the supernatant was filtered using a 0.45-μm syringe filter. LC-MS was performed on an Acquity UPLC BEH C18 column (1.7 μm, 2.1 mm × 100 mm; Waters, Milford, MA, USA) with a column temperature of 40 °C and a flow rate of 0.4 mL/min. The mobile phase was comprised of solvent A (0.1% formic acid in water) and solvent B (100% acetonitrile) with the following elution gradient maintained at 90% A for 4 min, reduced to 5% A over 10 min, maintained at 5% A for 1 min, increased to 90% A over 0.5 min, and maintained at 90% A for 1.5 min. The lower limit of quantification was 0.1 mg/L. The inter- and intra-assay coefficients of variation were <15%.

The population PK model was conducted based on non-linear mixed-effects modelling using NONMEM (version 7.4.1; ICON Development Solutions, Dublin, Ireland) and Pirana (version 2.9.7; Certara, Princeton, NJ, USA). The Xpose4 package (version 4.6.1; https://github.com/UUPharmacometrics/xpose4/releases (accessed on 1 March 2019)) in R (version 3.5.3; http://www.r-project.org (accessed on 1 March 2019)) was used to visualize and evaluate the models.

The plasma concentration-time profiles for meropenem were fitted to one-, two-, or three-compartment models using the first-order conditional estimation method with the interaction estimation option. Interindividual variability (IIV) of the PK parameters was evaluated using an exponential variance model assuming a log-normal distribution. Residual unexplained variability (RUV) was tested using an additive, exponential, and combined random error model. The model was selected based on a minimum objective function value (OFV), validity of the estimated relative standard error (RSE), shrinkage of PK parameters, and visual inspection of the goodness-of-fit plot. The likelihood ratio test was performed in the NONMEM program to assess statistical significance between the nested models. A decrease in the OFV of at least 3.84 was judged statistically significant for an added parameter (p value < 0.05, χ^2 distribution, degree of freedom = 1). For visual inspection, the goodness-of-fit plot was expressed as the observed concentrations vs. population predictions (PRED) or individual predictions (IPRED), and conditional weighted residuals (CWRES) vs. PRED.

To evaluate the influence of covariates on the meropenem PK parameters, the following potential covariates were tested: demographic variables (sex, age, weight, and height), ECMO-associated variables (during ECMO or weaned off of ECMO and ECMO flow rate [LPM, liters per minute]), CRRT-associated variables (use of CRRT, blood flow rate, CRRT 6 h prior to urine output, dialysate flow rate), complete blood count (absolute white blood cells, red blood cells, hemoglobin, and platelets), renal function (serum creatinine [SCr], blood urea nitrogen [BUN], creatinine clearance (CrCL) estimated via the Cockcroft-Gault equation, and eGFR estimated via the MDRD equation), liver function (alanine transaminase, aspartate aminotransferase, and total bilirubin), biomarkers of inflammation (C-reactive protein and procalcitonin), blood pressure, tympanic body temperature, and social variables (smoking status and alcohol consumption). In addition, to reflect the inherent correlation between patient status and improvement in critical illness between the ECMO-ON and ECMO-OFF groups, we tested the time since ECMO initiation and ECMO termination as an individual covariate. Most data were tested as time-varying covariates, except fixed variables, such as sex, age, and smoking status, which were considered time-independent.

Covariates were evaluated using linear, exponential, power, and proportional models based on the stepwise covariate modelling (SCM) process. If needed, the continuous covariates were centered on their median values. For forward selection, a p value < 0.05 (OFV reduction of >3.84) and for backward elimination, a $p < 0.01$ (OFV increase of >6.64) were considered to measure significance. The final covariate model selection was based on biological or clinical plausibility, RSE, shrinkage of PK parameters, a condition number of <1000, and visual improvement in the goodness-of-fit plot.

To evaluate the precision and robustness of the final PK model, an automated sampling importance resampling (SIR) algorithm (sampling = 5000, resampling = 1000, five iterations) and a prediction-corrected visual predictive check (pcVPC) were carried out using the Perl Speaks NONMEM toolkit version 4.9.0. (Uppsala University, Uppsala, Sweden) [18,19]. The medians with 95% confidence intervals for the replicates from the SIR algorithm were compared with the estimated PK parameters from the final model. Furthermore, the simulated pcVPC results with the 5th percentile, median, and 95th percentile curves were visually assessed.

Monte Carlo simulations were performed using the estimated PK parameters to assess the effect of the screened covariates on the predicted meropenem concentrations (n = 10,000). Intravenous intermittent infusion (II) over 20 min. and intravenous extended infusion (EI) over 3 h and 6 h were simulated by the following dosage regimens: 1 g q12h, 2 g q12h, 0.5 g q8h, 1 g q8h, and 2 g q8h over a 24-h period since the first meropenem administration. In addition, intravenous continuous infusion (CI) over 8 h (q8h) of 0.5, 1, and 2 g were simulated. The % fT > MIC was determined for each simulated subject by linear interpolation. The PTA was calculated by counting subjects achieving more than 40% fT > MIC and 100% fT > MIC; the dosage scenario that achieved PTA above 90% was considered to be efficient. The MIC, the clinical breakpoint for meropenem, that was used was 2 mg/L for susceptible strains and 8 mg/L for resistant strains according to EUCAST (ver. 10.0, Växjö, Sweden, valid from 1 January 2020).

Ethical Aspects

The study was approved by the Severance Hospital Institutional Review Board (approval number: 4-2014-0919) and conducted in accordance with the principles of the Declaration of Helsinki and national and institutional standards and was registered at Clinicaltrials.gov (NCT02581280). Written informed consent was obtained from the unconscious participants' legally acceptable representatives.

3. Results

Thirteen patients were included in our study, and eleven of them received V-A ECMO because of acute myocardial infarction (MI). Five patients received CRRT concomitantly among the six patients in the ECMO-ON group; two patients received CRRT among the nine patients in the ECMO-OFF group. Two patients were sampled repeatedly based on their ECMO status. The median values of age, weight, SCr, and APACHE II score were 55 years, 65.8 kg, 1.2 mg/dL, and 30, respectively, at the initiation of ECMO. The median value of eGFR was 70.4 mL/min/1.73 m^2, and the eGFR of all patients not receiving CRRT was above 30 mL/min/1.73 m^2 (Table 1).

Table 1. Demographic information and baseline characteristics of all enrolled patients.

ECMO	Patient No. *	Age Range (yr)	Sex	Wt (kg)	Ht (m)	Diagnosis	SCr (mg/dL)	CRRT	eGFR (mL/min/ 1.73 m^2)	APACHE II Score	Length of Hospital Stay (Days)
On	1	45–49	M	74.6	1.73	Acute MI	na #	yes	na #	34	15
	2	50–54	M	74.6	1.70	Acute MI,	na #	yes	na #	32	27
	3	50–54	M	82.9	1.68	Acute MI	na #	yes	na #	44	40
	4	55–59	F	69.9	1.64	Acute MI	na #	yes	na #	30	200
	5	70–74	M	93.3	1.70	Acute MI	na #	yes	na #	36	21
	6	50–59	M	53.1	1.68	Acute MI	1.06	no	76.5	29	36

Table 1. *Cont.*

ECMO	Patient No. *	Age Range (yr)	Sex	Wt (kg)	Ht (m)	Diagnosis	SCr (mg/dL)	CRRT	eGFR (mL/min/ 1.73 m^2)	APACHE II Score	Length of Hospital Stay (Days)
Off	4 *	55–59	F	67.4	1.64		1.2	no	49.6	30	200
	6 *	55–59	M	53.1	1.68		0.88	no	94.9	29	36
	7	50–54	F	48.2	1.46	Acute MI	na #	yes	na #	37	75
	8	75–79	M	53.9	1.60	Acute MI	na #	yes	na #	40	75
	9	45–49	M	61.1	1.72	Acute MI	1.3	no	64.3	22	21
	10	55–59	F	60.0	1.62	VF arrest	0.5	no	127.3	30	29
	11	55–59	M	77.5	1.68	Acute MI, VF arrest	2.0	no	36.5	28	37
	12	50–54	M	63.0	1.62	VF arrest	0.7	no	120.4	26	36
	13	65–69	M	67.4	1.68 §	Acute MI	1.3	no	60.3	14	23
		55 (53–58)		67.4 (57–74.6)	1.68 (1.63–1.70)		1.2 (0.7–1.56)		70.4 (57.6–101.3)	30 (28.5–35)	36 (25–57.5)

* The same number represents the same patient according to the ECMO status. § The mean value was used because data were missing. # Not listed because it is CRRT-dependent. ECMO, extracorporeal membrane oxygenation; CRRT, continuous renal replacement therapy; M, male; F, female; Wt, weight; Ht, height; SCr, serum creatinine; eGFR, estimated glomerular filtration rate according to Modification of Diet in Renal Disease Study equation; VF, ventricular fibrillation; MI, myocardial infarction; yr, year.

The time profile of meropenem plasma concentrations was best fitted by a two-compartment model with IIV on CL and peripheral volume of distribution (V2). The RUV was best explained by an exponential error model. After stepwise selection, the use of CRRT for CL was included in the final PK model; the CL of the patients receiving CRRT was lower than that of the patients not receiving CRRT (ΔOFV = 16.8, condition number = 164.5). As covariates, the use of ECMO and the time since ECMO initiation and ECMO termination were not selected by the SCM process, because they were not shown to be statistically significant and did not improve the goodness-of-fit of the model. The CrCL and eGFR were not selected for the same reason. The final PK model is described as follows.

$$\text{CL (L/h)} = 3.79 \times 0.44^{\text{CRRT}}; \quad (1)$$

where the use of CRRT = 1, no use of CRRT = 0

$$\text{V1 (L)} = 2.4 \quad (2)$$

$$\text{V2 (L)} = 8.56 \quad (3)$$

$$\text{Q (L/h)} = 21.3 \quad (4)$$

where V1 is the central volume of distribution and Q is the intercompartmental clearance.

The values of CL from Equation (1) were 3.79 L/h and 1.67 L/h in patients with CRRT and without CRRT, respectively. The parameter estimates and SIR results with 95% confidence intervals are presented in Table 2. All ETA shrinkage values were <40% in the final model. All parameters had acceptable RSE values, except for the IIV of V2. The goodness-of-fit plots are shown in Figure S1. Both population and individual predictions were distributed uniformly across the line of equality. The plots of CWRES vs. PRED did not show any trends. The pcVPC plot showed that approximately 10% of the observed data was positioned outside of the 5th to 95th percentiles of the predicted data, which suggested that the predictive performance of the final model was adequate (Figure 1).

Table 2. Parameter estimates of the base model and final model.

Parameter	Base Model	Final Model	
	Population Estimate (RSE)	Population Estimate (RSE)	SIR Median (2.5th–97.5th Percentile)
Fixed effects (θ)			
CL (L/h)	2.65 (32%)	3.79 (26%)	3.77 (2.69–5.37)
Central volume of distribution, V1 (L)	2.53 (21%)	2.4 (38%)	2.76 (0.59–4.84)
Peripheral volume of distribution, V2 (L)	9.61 (38%)	8.56 (22%)	8.36 (5.59–12.93)
Intercompartmental clearance, Q (L/h)	20.8 (9%)	21.3 (17%)	19.94 (9.37–33.41)
θ_{CRRT} on CL	-	0.44 (30%)	0.45 (0.29–0.62)
Random effects (% CV)			
Interindividual variability (ω^2)			
CL	69.4 (36%)	47.1 (49%)	49.2 (32.2–74.2)
V2	61 (103%)	44 (154%)	51.1 (7.7–108)
Residual unexplained variability (σ^2)	49.7 (18%)	47.3 (21%)	49.0 (40.9–60.2)

RSE, relative standard error; CV, coefficient of variation; SIR, sampling importance resampling.

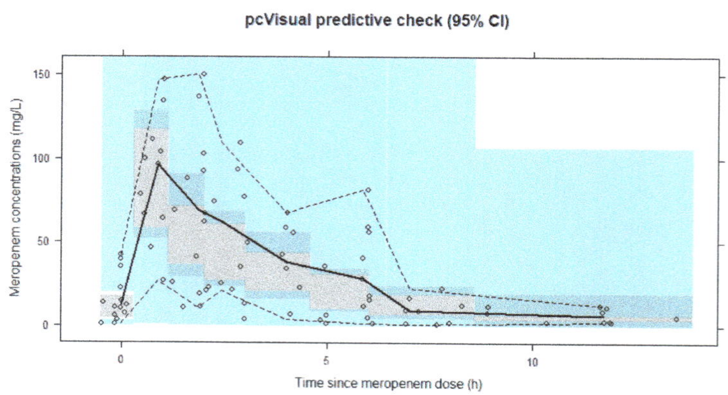

Figure 1. Prediction-corrected visual predictive check plot. The prediction-corrected visual predictive check plot shows that the 5th to 95th percentiles of the predicted data overlap most of the observed data based on time since meropenem dose. Open diamonds, plasma meropenem concentrations; solid line, median; lower and upper dashed lines, 5th and 95th percentiles of the observed data, respectively; shaded areas, 95% confidence intervals for simulated predicted median, 5th percentile, and 95th percentile constructed from 5000 simulated data sets of individuals from the original data set.

The final PK model was used for the Monte Carlo simulation (n = 10,000), and the simulated PTA vs. MIC profiles for various dosage scenarios are shown in Table S1. Almost all dosage scenarios were sufficient to achieve a PTA above 90% at 40% fT > MIC, regardless of the administration frequency, route (II, EI, or CI), pathogen susceptibility, or use of CRRT. Target PTAs could be more readily achieved with EI or CI than with II; when comparing EI over 3 h with EI over 6 h, there was little noticeable difference in achieving target PTAs. However, when more aggressive treatment was needed (i.e., PTA above 90% at 100% fT > MIC), achieving the target PTA was difficult in the simulated scenarios using II.

The recommended dosage regimens are shown in Table 3. Whether on ECMO or not, the standard doses of meropenem in patients with normal kidney function (1–2 g q8h II) and those in patients receiving CRRT (1 g q12h II or 0.5 g q8h II) were sufficient to cover both susceptible (MIC = 2 mg/L) and resistant (MIC = 8 mg/L) pathogens. Moreover, lower doses (0.5 g q8h for patients with normal kidney function and 0.5 g q8h for patients during CRRT) can also be recommended via EI or CI. If more aggressive treatment is needed, EI or CI is generally recommended. In patients not receiving CRRT, 2 g q8h EI over 6 h or CI is recommended against resistant pathogens. When the patients receiving CRRT require aggressive treatment against resistant pathogens, the minimum recommended dose is 1 g q8h EI or 0.5–1 g q8h CI.

Table 3. Recommended dose regimen for meropenem.

Target	Normal Therapy (40% *f*T > MIC)		More Aggressive Therapy (100% *f*T > MIC)	
	For Susceptible Pathogens (MIC = 2 mg/L)	**For Resistant Pathogens (MIC = 8 mg/L)**	**For Susceptible Pathogens (MIC = 2 mg/L)**	**For resistant Pathogens (MIC = 8 mg/L)**
without CRRT	**1–2 g q8h II** 0.5 g q8h EIs or CI	**1–2 g q8h II** 0.5 g q8h EIs or CI	1–2 g q8h EIs or CI	2 g q8h EI over 6 h or CI
with CRRT	**1 g q12h II** **0.5 g q8h II** 0.5 g q8h EIs or CI	**1 g q12h II** **0.5 g q8h II** 0.5 g q8h EIs or CI	**1 g q12h II** **0.5 g q8h II** 0.5 g q8h EIs or CI	1 g q8h EIs 0.5–1 g q8h CI

The bold doses indicate the standard dosage regimens in the manuscript. II, intravenous intermittent infusion over 20 min; EIs, intravenous extended infusions over 3 h and 6 h; EI, intravenous extended infusion; CI, intravenous continuous infusion; CRRT, continuous renal replacement therapy.

4. Discussion

This prospective cohort study was designed to develop a population PK model for meropenem in patients receiving V-A ECMO, and to explore the appropriate dosage regimen of meropenem by analyzing the probability of target attainment using Monte Carlo simulations. In our final PK model, a two-compartment model best fit the time course of plasma meropenem concentrations. This study revealed that the use of ECMO did not have a significant impact on the PK of meropenem. Meanwhile, meropenem CL was 0.44 times lower in patients with CRRT than in patients without CRRT (kidney function >30 mL/min/1.73 m^2); however, the contributing factors related to CRRT did not help improve the final PK model. As the result of PTA assessment, the standard dose of meropenem was deemed sufficient to cover both susceptible and resistant pathogens in patients receiving CRRT (1 g q12h II or 0.5 g q8h II) or in patients with preserved renal function (1–2 g q8h II) regardless of ECMO. However, if aggressive treatment was needed, EI over 3–6 h or CI instead of II or incremental dosing was appropriate. These results can help provide a clinically appropriate dosage regimen for meropenem in patients receiving both V-A ECMO and CRRT.

In our study, CL decreased in patients receiving CRRT regardless of V-A ECMO treatment. Meropenem is reported to be excreted mainly by the kidneys, and renal function indices, such as eGFR estimated by the MDRD Study equation and CrCL estimated via the Cockcroft-Gault equation, were also found to have a positive relationship with meropenem CL [16,17]. We assessed the relationship between renal function and meropenem CL in the univariate analysis among non-CRRT patients. However, renal function indices were excluded as covariates because they did not improve robustness of the PK model, which differed from CRRT added to CL as a covariate. This result may be explained by the small number of patients enrolled in the present study and the fact that almost all included patients without CRRT had eGFR > 30 mL/min/1.73 m^2. In our final PK model, eGFR was not selected as a covariate; however, this does not indicate that dose adjustments according to estimated renal function are not required.

No covariates, including the use of V-A ECMO, affected the Vd of meropenem in our PK model. Patients undergoing V-A ECMO generally need vigorous volume support including resuscitation fluid and transfusion, owing to the initial circuit priming volume and their hemodynamic instability [20]. This could lead to increased circulating volume, but meropenem is relatively hydrophilic, and has low protein binding affinity [21], thus, its sequestration on the ECMO surface may not be high. Because of these properties, V-A ECMO may have little effect on the Vd of meropenem despite the larger circulating volume. Other investigators have also reported similar results, in that the use of ECMO did not influence the Vd of meropenem [16,17].

Moreover, our findings showed that V-A ECMO did not significantly alter the PK of meropenem, consistent with the results of previous PK studies in patients receiving meropenem during both V-A and V-V ECMO [16,22]. Hanberg et al. studied population PKs of meropenem in 10 patients and they reported that standard dosing is enough during ECMO treatment [16]. Another case-control study said that PK changes of β-lactam antibiotics are not significant in patients on ECMO [22]. Other β-lactam antibiotics, which have similar pharmacokinetic characteristics reported conflicting results. One study reported larger dose is necessary for cefepime in patients receiving ECMO [23], as well as the previous study of cefpirome [24]. On the contrary, ECMO did not affect the PKs of ceftriaxone and standard dosing was sufficient [25]. Such high hydrophilic antibiotics showed different changes in PK, and individual PK studies of each antibiotic is necessary. A recent review suggested that the PK change in ECMO patients was more reflective of critical illness than the ECMO device [14]. Therefore, the PK changes observed for meropenem might be affected not by ECMO use, but by critical illness, which includes renal and hepatic hypoperfusion, hypoxia, and systemic inflammation. Thus, therapeutic drug monitoring is recommended [13,14].

The optimal PK/pharmacodynamics (PD) index to assess the bactericidal activity of meropenem is the percentage of the time in which the total drug concentration is above the MIC of a pathogen during the antibiotic dosing interval (fT > MIC) [26–29]. A fT > MIC of 40% is frequently used for maximum bactericidal effect, as reported by a recent in silico study [29,30], but this is still controversial. Several clinical studies recommend therapeutic drug monitoring to ensure 100% fT > MIC for beta-lactams in critically ill patients [31–33]. Other reports have suggested that PK targets maintain plasma beta-lactam concentrations of more than 4 times the MIC ($fT > 4 \times$ MIC) for the optimal treatment of severe infections [34,35].

In our study, the current standard dosage recommendation was still effective, but EI or CI provided better PTA and either infusion is recommended when aggressive treatment is needed. The clinical benefits of prolonged administration of beta-lactams, which display time-dependent activity, have previously been shown [36–39]. One issue in the prolonged administration of meropenem is time-and temperature-dependent degradation [40–42]. However, data from several studies have suggested that >90% meropenem remains in vitro after 5–6 h at room temperature [40,42]. Also recent evidence suggests that meropenem degradation during CI is insignificant at the end of a 12-h dosing interval at room temperature [43]. Therefore, we suggest that EI over 3 h or 6 h would be better than CI if the PK/PD target were to be attained, since meropenem stability during infusion would not be a concern.

To the best of our knowledge, this study is the first to investigate the PK changes in meropenem by comparing patients during V-A ECMO with those weaned off of V-A ECMO and to suggest the optimal dosage of meropenem according to various scenarios between ECMO and CRRT. However, this study was limited by the relatively small sample size conducted in a single center and, therefore, the data may not have provided robust PK parameter estimates. We attempted to use the ECMO-OFF group as a control to directly compare the effects on ECMO and reduce IIV between the control and intervention groups. However, only two patients could be included in both the ECMO-ON and ECMO-OFF groups because meropenem is not a first-line antibiotic according to our hospital protocol. Finally, our PK model was restricted to patients receiving V-A ECMO and CRRT, which is merely one mode of ECMO and CRRT. Therefore, the applicability of our results to all modes of ECMO is limited.

5. Conclusions

In conclusion, we established a PK/PD model for meropenem in patients receiving ECMO. Moreover, we suggest optimized dosage regimens to provide adequate bactericidal activity. The standard dosage regimen (1–2 g q8h II) was sufficient to treat both susceptible and resistant pathogens. If more aggressive therapy is needed, a dose increment or EI over

3–6 h is recommended. These findings will contribute for the considerations of meropenem dosing in patients receiving V-A ECMO.

Supplementary Materials: The following supporting information can be downloaded at: https://www.mdpi.com/article/10.3390/jcm11226621/s1, Figure S1: Goodness-of-fit plots of the final population model for meropenem; Table S1: Probability of target attainment for 10,000 simulated subjects given meropenem.

Author Contributions: S.K., J.W. and M.J.C. designed the study, performed the population. PK analysis, interpreted the results of the analysis, and draft the manuscript. J.W. and M.J.C. supervised the design, conducted the study, and revised the manuscript. S.K., S.Y., J.H., J.Y.J. and K.L.M. collected the blood sample and patient data. S.Y. assisted technical PK modelling and reviewed the manuscript. All authors have read and agreed to the published version of the manuscript.

Funding: This work was supported by a grant (No. 2020R1F1A1070549) from the National Research Foundation (NRF) of Korea, funded by the Korean government (Ministry of Science, ICT & Future Planning), and Gachon University research fund of 2020 (GCU-2020-202005400001).

Institutional Review Board Statement: The study was approved by the Severance Hospital Institutional Review Board (approval number: 4-2014-0919) and was registered at Clinicaltrials.gov (NCT02581280). Written informed consent was obtained from the unconscious participants' legally acceptable representatives

Informed Consent Statement: Informed consent was obtained from all subjects involved in the study.

Acknowledgments: We would like to acknowledge all of the staff of the cardiac intensive care unit of Severance Hospital for their practical support and patient care. They played a crucial role in the successful completion of this study.

Conflicts of Interest: The authors declare no conflict of interest.

References

1. Ouweneel, D.M.; Schotborgh, J.V.; Limpens, J.; Sjauw, K.D.; Engström, A.E.; Lagrand, W.K.; Cherpanath, T.G.V.; Driessen, A.H.G.; de Mol, B.; Henriques, J.P.S. Extracorporeal life support during cardiac arrest and cardiogenic shock: A systematic review and meta-analysis. *Intensive Care Med.* **2016**, *42*, 1922–1934. [CrossRef] [PubMed]
2. Thiagarajan, R.R.; Barbaro, R.P.; Rycus, P.T.; McMullan, D.M.; Conrad, S.A.; Fortenberry, J.D.; Paden, M.L. Extracorporeal Life Support Organization Registry International Report 2016. *ASAIO J.* **2017**, *63*, 60–67. [CrossRef] [PubMed]
3. Loforte, A.; Marinelli, G.; Musumeci, F.; Folesani, G.; Pilato, E.; Martin Suarez, S.; Montalto, A.; Lilla Della Monica, P.; Grigioni, F.; Frascaroli, G.; et al. Extracorporeal membrane oxygenation support in refractory cardiogenic shock: Treatment strategies and analysis of risk factors. *Artif. Organs* **2014**, *38*, E129–E141. [CrossRef] [PubMed]
4. Kim, H.S.; Park, S.; Ko, H.H.; Ha, S.O.; Lee, S.H.; Kim, Y.K. Different characteristics of bloodstream infection during venoarterial and venovenous extracorporeal membrane oxygenation in adult patients. *Sci. Rep.* **2021**, *11*, 9498. [CrossRef] [PubMed]
5. Aubron, C.; Cheng, A.C.; Pilcher, D.; Leong, T.; Magrin, G.; Cooper, D.J.; Scheinkestel, C.; Pellegrino, V. Infections acquired by adults who receive extracorporeal membrane oxygenation: Risk factors and outcome. *Infect. Control. Hosp. Epidemiol.* **2013**, *34*, 24–30. [CrossRef]
6. Sherwin, J.; Heath, T.; Watt, K. Pharmacokinetics and Dosing of Anti-infective Drugs in Patients on Extracorporeal Membrane Oxygenation: A Review of the Current Literature. *Clin. Ther.* **2016**, *38*, 1976–1994. [CrossRef]
7. Hahn, J.; Choi, J.H.; Chang, M.J. Pharmacokinetic changes of antibiotic, antiviral, antituberculosis and antifungal agents during extracorporeal membrane oxygenation in critically ill adult patients. *J. Clin. Pharm. Ther.* **2017**, *42*, 661–671. [CrossRef]
8. Ha, M.A.; Sieg, A.C. Evaluation of Altered Drug Pharmacokinetics in Critically Ill Adults Receiving Extracorporeal Membrane Oxygenation. *Pharmacotherapy* **2017**, *37*, 221–235. [CrossRef]
9. Shekar, K.; Roberts, J.A.; McDonald, C.I.; Ghassabian, S.; Anstey, C.; Wallis, S.C.; Mullany, D.V.; Fung, Y.L.; Fraser, J.F. Protein-bound drugs are prone to sequestration in the extracorporeal membrane oxygenation circuit: Results from an ex vivo study. *Crit. Care* **2015**, *19*, 164. [CrossRef]
10. Shekar, K.; Roberts, J.A.; McDonald, C.I.; Fisquet, S.; Barnett, A.G.; Mullany, D.V.; Ghassabian, S.; Wallis, S.C.; Fung, Y.L.; Smith, M.T.; et al. Sequestration of drugs in the circuit may lead to therapeutic failure during extracorporeal membrane oxygenation. *Crit. Care* **2012**, *16*, R194. [CrossRef]
11. Mousavi, S.; Levcovich, B.; Mojtahedzadeh, M. A systematic review on pharmacokinetic changes in critically ill patients: Role of extracorporeal membrane oxygenation. *DARU* **2011**, *19*, 312–321.

12. Thiele, H.; Ohman, E.M.; de Waha-Thiele, S.; Zeymer, U.; Desch, S. Management of cardiogenic shock complicating myocardial infarction: An update 2019. *Eur. Heart J.* **2019**, *40*, 2671–2683. [CrossRef]
13. Cheng, V.; Abdul-Aziz, M.H.; Roberts, J.A.; Shekar, K. Optimising drug dosing in patients receiving extracorporeal membrane oxygenation. *J. Thorac. Dis.* **2018**, *10*, S629–S641. [CrossRef]
14. Abdul-Aziz, M.H.; Roberts, J.A. Antibiotic dosing during extracorporeal membrane oxygenation: Does the system matter? *Curr. Opin. Anaesthesiol.* **2020**, *33*, 71–82. [CrossRef]
15. Hahn, J.; Min, K.L.; Kang, S.; Yang, S.; Park, M.S.; Wi, J.; Chang, M.J. Population Pharmacokinetics and Dosing Optimization of Piperacillin-Tazobactam in Critically Ill Patients on Extracorporeal Membrane Oxygenation and the Influence of Concomitant Renal Replacement Therapy. *Microbiol. Spectr.* **2021**, *9*, e0063321. [CrossRef]
16. Hanberg, P.; Öbrink-Hansen, K.; Thorsted, A.; Bue, M.; Tøttrup, M.; Friberg, L.E.; Hardlei, T.F.; Søballe, K.; Gjedsted, J. Population Pharmacokinetics of Meropenem in Plasma and Subcutis from Patients on Extracorporeal Membrane Oxygenation Treatment. *Antimicrob. Agents Chemother.* **2018**, *62*, e02390-17. [CrossRef]
17. Shekar, K.; Fraser, J.F.; Taccone, F.S.; Welch, S.; Wallis, S.C.; Mullany, D.V.; Lipman, J.; Roberts, J.A. The combined effects of extracorporeal membrane oxygenation and renal replacement therapy on meropenem pharmacokinetics: A matched cohort study. *Crit. Care* **2014**, *18*, 565. [CrossRef]
18. Post, T.M.; Freijer, J.I.; Ploeger, B.A.; Danhof, M. Extensions to the visual predictive check to facilitate model performance evaluation. *J. Pharmacokinet. Pharmacodyn.* **2008**, *35*, 185–202. [CrossRef]
19. Dosne, A.G.; Bergstrand, M.; Karlsson, M.O. An automated sampling importance resampling procedure for estimating parameter uncertainty. *J. Pharmacokinet. Pharmacodyn.* **2017**, *44*, 509–520. [CrossRef]
20. Shekar, K.; Fraser, J.F.; Smith, M.T.; Roberts, J.A. Pharmacokinetic changes in patients receiving extracorporeal membrane oxygenation. *J. Crit. Care* **2012**, *27*, 741.e9–741.e18. [CrossRef]
21. Wishart, D.S.; Feunang, Y.D.; Guo, A.C.; Lo, E.J.; Marcu, A.; Grant, J.R.; Sajed, T.; Johnson, D.; Li, C.; Sayeeda, Z.; et al. DrugBank 5.0: A major update to the DrugBank database for 2018. *Nucleic Acids Res.* **2018**, *46*, D1074–D1082. [CrossRef] [PubMed]
22. Donadello, K.; Antonucci, E.; Cristallini, S.; Roberts, J.A.; Beumier, M.; Scolletta, S.; Jacobs, F.; Rondelet, B.; de Backer, D.; Vincent, J.L.; et al. β-Lactam pharmacokinetics during extracorporeal membrane oxygenation therapy: A case-control study. *Int. J. Antimicrob. Agents* **2015**, *45*, 278–282. [CrossRef] [PubMed]
23. Kois, A.K.; Gluck, J.A.; Nicolau, D.P.; Kuti, J.L. Pharmacokinetics and Time above the MIC Exposure of Cefepime in Critically Ill Patients Receiving Extracorporeal Membrane Oxygenation (ECMO). *Int. J. Antimicrob. Agents* **2022**, *60*, 106603. [CrossRef] [PubMed]
24. Kang, S.; Jang, J.Y.; Hahn, J.; Kim, D.; Lee, J.Y.; Min, K.L.; Yang, S.; Wi, J.; Chang, M.J. Dose Optimization of Cefpirome Based on Population Pharmacokinetics and Target Attainment during Extracorporeal Membrane Oxygenation. *Antimicrob. Agents Chemother.* **2020**, *64*, e00249-20. [CrossRef] [PubMed]
25. Cheng, V.; Abdul-Aziz, M.H.; Burrows, F.; Buscher, H.; Cho, Y.J.; Corley, A.; Gilder, E.; Kim, H.S.; Lim, S.Y.; McGuinness, S.; et al. Population Pharmacokinetics and Dosing Simulations of Ceftriaxone in Critically Ill Patients Receiving Extracorporeal Membrane Oxygenation (An ASAP ECMO Study). *Clin. Pharmacokinet.* **2022**, *61*, 847–856. [CrossRef]
26. Craig, W.A. Interrelationship between pharmacokinetics and pharmacodynamics in determining dosage regimens for broad-spectrum cephalosporins. *Diagn. Microbiol. Infect. Dis.* **1995**, *22*, 89–96. [CrossRef]
27. Nielsen, E.I.; Cars, O.; Friberg, L.E. Pharmacokinetic/pharmacodynamic (PK/PD) indices of antibiotics predicted by a semimechanistic PKPD model: A step toward model-based dose optimization. *Antimicrob. Agents Chemother.* **2011**, *55*, 4619–4630. [CrossRef]
28. Onufrak, N.J.; Forrest, A.; Gonzalez, D. Pharmacokinetic and Pharmacodynamic Principles of Anti-infective Dosing. *Clin. Ther.* **2016**, *38*, 1930–1947. [CrossRef]
29. Kristoffersson, A.N.; David-Pierson, P.; Parrott, N.J.; Kuhlmann, O.; Lave, T.; Friberg, L.E.; Nielsen, E.I. Simulation-Based Evaluation of PK/PD Indices for Meropenem Across Patient Groups and Experimental Designs. *Pharm. Res.* **2016**, *33*, 1115–1125. [CrossRef]
30. Drusano, G.L. Prevention of resistance: A goal for dose selection for antimicrobial agents. *Clin. Infect. Dis.* **2003**, *36*, S42–S50. [CrossRef]
31. Li, C.; Du, X.; Kuti, J.L.; Nicolau, D.P. Clinical pharmacodynamics of meropenem in patients with lower respiratory tract infections. *Antimicrob. Agents Chemother.* **2007**, *51*, 1725–1730. [CrossRef]
32. Roberts, J.A.; Paul, S.K.; Akova, M.; Bassetti, M.; De Waele, J.J.; Dimopoulos, G.; Kaukonen, K.M.; Koulenti, D.; Martin, C.; Montravers, P.; et al. DALI: Defining antibiotic levels in intensive care unit patients: Are current β-lactam antibiotic doses sufficient for critically ill patients? *Clin. Infect. Dis.* **2014**, *58*, 1072–1083. [CrossRef]
33. Huttner, A.; Harbarth, S.; Hope, W.W.; Lipman, J.; Roberts, J.A. Therapeutic drug monitoring of the β-lactam antibiotics: What is the evidence and which patients should we be using it for? *J. Antimicrob. Chemother.* **2015**, *70*, 3178–3183. [CrossRef]
34. Roberts, J.A.; Ulldemolins, M.; Roberts, M.S.; McWhinney, B.; Ungerer, J.; Paterson, D.L.; Lipman, J. Therapeutic drug monitoring of beta-lactams in critically ill patients: Proof of concept. *Int. J. Antimicrob. Agents* **2010**, *36*, 332–339. [CrossRef]
35. Mouton, J.W.; Vinks, A.A. Continuous infusion of beta-lactams. *Curr. Opin. Crit. Care* **2007**, *13*, 598–606. [CrossRef]
36. Mohd Hafiz, A.A.; Staatz, C.E.; Kirkpatrick, C.M.; Lipman, J.; Roberts, J.A. Continuous infusion vs. bolus dosing: Implications for beta-lactam antibiotics. *Minerva Anestesiol.* **2012**, *78*, 94–104.

37. Bauer, K.A.; West, J.E.; O'Brien, J.M.; Goff, D.A. Extended-infusion cefepime reduces mortality in patients with Pseudomonas aeruginosa infections. *Antimicrob. Agents Chemother.* **2013**, *57*, 2907–2912. [CrossRef]
38. Kuti, J.L.; Nightingale, C.H.; Knauft, R.F.; Nicolau, D.P. Pharmacokinetic properties and stability of continuous-infusion meropenem in adults with cystic fibrosis. *Clin. Ther.* **2004**, *26*, 493–501. [CrossRef]
39. Roberts, J.A.; Kirkpatrick, C.M.; Roberts, M.S.; Robertson, T.A.; Dalley, A.J.; Lipman, J. Meropenem dosing in critically ill patients with sepsis and without renal dysfunction: Intermittent bolus versus continuous administration? Monte Carlo dosing simulations and subcutaneous tissue distribution. *J. Antimicrob. Chemother.* **2009**, *64*, 142–150. [CrossRef]
40. Berthoin, K.; Le Duff, C.S.; Marchand-Brynaert, J.; Carryn, S.; Tulkens, P.M. Stability of meropenem and doripenem solutions for administration by continuous infusion. *J. Antimicrob. Chemother.* **2010**, *65*, 1073–1075. [CrossRef]
41. Patel, P.R.; Cook, S.E. Stability of meropenem in intravenous solutions. *Am. J. Health Syst. Pharm.* **1997**, *54*, 412–421. [CrossRef] [PubMed]
42. Viaene, E.; Chanteux, H.; Servais, H.; Mingeot-Leclercq, M.P.; Tulkens, P.M. Comparative stability studies of antipseudomonal beta-lactams for potential administration through portable elastomeric pumps (home therapy for cystic fibrosis patients) and motor-operated syringes (intensive care units). *Antimicrob. Agents Chemother.* **2002**, *46*, 2327–2332. [CrossRef] [PubMed]
43. Venugopalan, V.; Manigaba, K.; Borgert, S.J.; Cope, J.; Peloquin, C.A.; Klinker, K.P. Training a Drug to Do New Tricks: Insights on Stability of Meropenem Administered as a Continuous Infusion. *Microbiol. Insights* **2018**, *11*, 1178636118804549. [CrossRef] [PubMed]

Journal of
Clinical Medicine

MDPI

Article

Invasiveness of Ventilation Therapy Is Associated to Prevalence of Secondary Bacterial and Fungal Infections in Critically Ill COVID-19 Patients

Marie Louise de Hesselle [1], Stefan Borgmann [2], Siegbert Rieg [3], Jörg Janne Vehreshild [4,5,6], Christoph D. Spinner [7,8], Carolin E. M. Koll [5,6], Martin Hower [9], Melanie Stecher [5,6], Daniel Ebert [1], Frank Hanses [10,†], Julia Schumann [1,*,†] and on behalf of the LEOSS Study Group [‡]

1 University Clinic and Outpatient Clinic for Anesthesiology and Operative Intensive Care, University Medicine Halle (Saale), 06112 Halle (Saale), Germany
2 Department of Infectious Diseases and Infection Control, Ingolstadt Hospital, 85049 Ingolstadt, Germany
3 Department of Medicine II, University of Freiburg, 79106 Freiburg, Germany
4 Department II of Internal Medicine, Hematology and Oncology, Goethe University Frankfurt, 60323 Frankfurt, Germany
5 Department I of Internal Medicine, Center for Integrated Oncology Aachen Bonn Cologne Duesseldorf, Faculty of Medicine and University Hospital Cologne, University of Cologne, 50931 Cologne, Germany
6 German Center for Infection Research (DZIF), Partner Site Bonn-Cologne, 50937 Cologne, Germany
7 Department of Internal Medicine II, University Hospital Rechts Der Isar, School of Medicine, Technical University of Munich, 81675 Munich, Germany
8 German Center for Infection Research (DZIF), 38106 Brunswick, Germany
9 Department of Pneumology, Infectious Diseases, Internal Medicine and Intensive Care, Klinikum Dortmund GmbH, 44137 Dortmund, Germany
10 Emergency Department and Department for Infection Control and Infectious Diseases, University Hospital Regensburg, 93053 Regensburg, Germany
* Correspondence: julia.schumann@uk-halle.de
† These authors contributed equally to this work.
‡ Membership of LEOSS study group is provided in the Acknowledgments.

Citation: de Hesselle, M.L.; Borgmann, S.; Rieg, S.; Vehreshild, J.J.; Spinner, C.D.; Koll, C.E.M.; Hower, M.; Stecher, M.; Ebert, D.; Hanses, F.; et al. Invasiveness of Ventilation Therapy Is Associated to Prevalence of Secondary Bacterial and Fungal Infections in Critically Ill COVID-19 Patients. *J. Clin. Med.* **2022**, *11*, 5239. https://doi.org/10.3390/jcm11175239

Academic Editors: Luca Brazzi and Giorgia Montrucchio

Received: 5 August 2022
Accepted: 2 September 2022
Published: 5 September 2022

Publisher's Note: MDPI stays neutral with regard to jurisdictional claims in published maps and institutional affiliations.

Abstract: Superinfections are a fundamental critical care problem, and their significance in severe COVID-19 cases needs to be determined. This study analyzed data from the Lean European Open Survey on SARS-CoV-2-Infected Patients (LEOSS) cohort focusing on intensive care patients. A retrospective analysis of patient data from 840 cases of COVID-19 with critical courses demonstrated that co-infections were frequently present and were primarily of nosocomial origin. Furthermore, our analysis showed that invasive therapy procedures accompanied an increased risk for healthcare-associated infections. Non-ventilated ICU patients were rarely affected by secondary infections. The risk of infection, however, increased even when non-invasive ventilation was used. A further, significant increase in infection rates was seen with the use of invasive ventilation and even more so with extracorporeal membrane oxygenation (ECMO) therapy. The marked differences among ICU techniques used for the treatment of COVID-19-induced respiratory failure in terms of secondary infection risk profile should be taken into account for the optimal management of critically ill COVID-19 patients, as well as for adequate antimicrobial therapy.

Keywords: COVID-19; SARS-CoV-2; multidrug-resistant pathogens; bacterial infections; fungal infections; secondary infections; intensive care medicine; ventilation; ECMO

1. Introduction

COVID-19, a pulmonary disease from an infection with the single-stranded RNA virus SARS-CoV-2, has evolved into a global pandemic since March 2020. Clinical manifestation is highly variable. Asymptomatic courses, mild respiratory diseases, severe pneumonia, and severe organ dysfunction that can be accompanied by shock and death have been described [1–6]. A certain proportion of patients develop an increased respiratory rate (>30/min), a decrease in oxygen saturation with hypoxemia, and respiratory insufficiency, which requires intensive care, usually due to dyspnea [3–7].

During the course of the pandemic, specific therapies for COVID-19 have been developed. However, the corresponding drugs should be applied within the first days after infection [8]. Relative risk reduction with respect to hospitalization or adverse outcome by the administration of antivirals or neutralizing monoclonal antibodies was described with the initiation of therapy at 3 to a maximum of 6 days after symptom onset [8]. Therefore, in an intensive care unit (ICU), only supportive treatment options are available to alleviate symptoms. In severe respiratory failure, intubation and invasive ventilation is the standard therapy in clinical practice [9]. It is a life-saving measure and usually ensures a safe airway and sufficient oxygenation, along with carbon dioxide elimination [9]. Early intubation counteracts the progressive deterioration of lung function due to increased respiratory stress [4,6]. It has also been reported that the critical delay of intubation in the event of failure of non-invasive ventilation options is associated with a poorer prognosis [4,6]. However, invasive ventilation may be the cause of ventilator-associated lung injury [6,7,9]. In addition, the safe airway required for invasive ventilation can promote serious, even lethal, infections [10]. The scientific literature, therefore, also contains reports recommending the avoidance of intubation as long as it is not essential [11].

Patients with viral infections are known to be predisposed to secondary infections [12–16]. In particular, bacteria may benefit from viral infections, and even those that are normally harmless could turn into opportunistic pathogens. The viral facilitation of bacterial pathogenesis is based on complex and multifactorial processes that, ultimately, promote bacterial adherence, disrupt epithelial layers, lead to the displacement of commensal bacteria, and subvert the host immune response [16]. There are multiple reports associating SARS-CoV-2 with co-infections of, primarily, bacterial but also fungal origin. The most common bacterial microorganisms in respiratory cultures from COVID-19 patients are *Pseudomonas aeruginosa*, *Klebsiella* species, *Staphylococcus aureus*, *Escherichia coli*, and *Stenotrophomonas maltophilia* [13,14]. The main fungal pathogens identified are *Aspergillus* and *Candida* species, but there are also reports of secondary infections with *Mucormycetes*, *Histoplasma* spp, *Cryptococcus* spp, and *Pneumocystis jirovecii* [12]. Alarmingly, such secondary infections have been linked to a severe clinical course with possible poor outcome [15,16].

Infections are a common problem in ICUs. A critical condition, an impaired immune response, and invasive treatments (i.e., mechanical ventilation and catheterization) all pose risk factors for nosocomial infections [10,17–21]. It is of concern that secondary infections in viral diseases of the respiratory tract, such as influenza, have been described as causes of morbidity and mortality [22–25]. However, the prevalence and clinical impact of healthcare-associated infections of bacterial or fungal nature in COVID-19 patients treated in ICUs is not well-understood and constitutes a serious knowledge gap. There is also insufficient knowledge on whether bacterial colonialization present on admission impacts disease severity and outcome. More data on community-acquired colonializations, as well as nosocomial infections in ICUs, are needed to optimize the management and treatment of the most severe COVID-19 cases. This could not only help to save lives but also to improve antimicrobial stewardship [26–29].

The aim of the present study is to unravel the prevalence of community-acquired colonializations with multidrug-resistant bacteria, as well as healthcare-associated secondary bacterial and fungal infections, in critically ill COVID-19 patients treated at an ICU. The primary objective was to determine whether (i) there is an association between a patient's infection status and the ventilation therapy used and whether (ii) co-infections are related to mortality. The secondary objectives are to examine the frequency of use and the clinical benefit of antimicrobial therapy in critically ill COVID-19 patients.

2. Materials and Methods

2.1. Patient Cohort

This study analyzed patient data from the Lean European Open Survey on SARS-CoV-2-Infected Patients (LEOSS) cohort [30]. The LEOSS project represents a non-interventional, multicenter network that aims at addressing the lack of in-depth knowledge on the epidemiology and clinical course of COVID-19. Established in March 2020, the LEOSS registry encloses data mainly on hospitalized COVID-19 patients. In the LEOSS protocol, patients can be included via PCR confirmed diagnosis or rapid antigen tests as an acceptable alternative. Detailed information on LEOSS can be found on the project's website (https://leoss.net, accessed date: 5 August 2022). The study was registered at the German Clinical Trials Register (DRKS, No S00021145).

Clinical data are reported in an electronic case report form (eCRF) using the online platform ClinicalSurveys.net, which was developed by the University Hospital of Cologne (UHC), Germany, and is hosted by QuestBack, Oslo, Norway, on servers of the UHC [31]. Anonymized patient data are added to the LEOSS registry retrospectively at the end of the acute treatment setting, i.e., when either the treatment is completed or the patient has died. In order to ensure anonymity in all steps of the analysis process, an individual LEOSS Scientific Use File (SUF) was created, which is based on the LEOSS Public Use File (PUF) principles described in Jakob et al. [31]. Re-identification is prevented by vertical (categorical assessment of numerical variables) and horizontal data aggregation (data aggregation within the phases of disease). Categorization is based on four phases, which can be roughly characterized as asymptomatic or mild symptoms (uncomplicated phase), need for oxygen supplementation (complicated phase), need for critical care (critical phase), and the recovery phase. A detailed description of the clinical phases as defined in the LEOSS registry, as well as of the recorded data items, can be found on the project's website (https://leoss.net; accessed on 4 August 2022) and in [32].

2.2. Study Design

This analysis included data of 840 patients who were documented by a LEOSS partner site between 23 March 2020 and 12 October 2020 due to COVID-19 disease diagnosed and treated between February 2020 and October 2020. Only patients who reached the critical phase according to the definitions of the LEOSS database [32] during the course of their COVID-19 disease were included in the analysis. The onset of the critical phase was declared if at least one of the following criteria was present: need for catecholamines, life-threatening cardiac arrhythmia, need for unplanned mechanical ventilation (invasive or non-invasive), prolongation (>24 h) of planned mechanical ventilation, liver failure with Quick <50% or INR >3.5, a qSOFA score of $\geq$2, or acute renal failure with need of dialysis. Dedicated intensive care data items were developed by a working group of specialized intensive care physicians (LEOSS Intensive Care Group) and implemented in the LEOSS registry. From this set, the following data items were analyzed: (i) the colonialization status of the patients with regard to multidrug-resistant pathogens at baseline, i.e., day of positive SARS-CoV-2 diagnosis (multidrug-resistant, Gram-negative bacteria (3MRGN/4MRGN), methicillin-resistant *Staphylococcus aureus* (MRSA), and vancomycin-resistant enterococci (VRE)), as well as bacterial and fungal superinfections in the critical phase; (ii) the ventilation treatments performed (non-invasive ventilation, invasive ventilation, or extracorporeal membrane oxygenation (ECMO)); (iii) the medications used; and (iv) the outcome (recovery or death). 3MRGN and 4MRGN are enterobacteriaceae, *Pseudomonas aeruginosa*, and *Acinetobacter baumannii* exhibiting resistance to three or four of these antibiotics or antibiotic groups: piperacillin, carbapenems, quinolones, and cephalosporins of the third generation. Two endpoints were defined: (i) the prevalence of community-acquired colonializations and healthcare-associated secondary infections in patients in need of or receiving a specific ventilation therapy (non-invasive ventilation, invasive ventilation, or ECMO) and (ii) the effect of community-acquired colonializations and healthcare-associated secondary infections on patient outcome.

2.3. Statistical Analysis

All data were presented as categorical variables (numbers and percentages). To compare categorical variables, Pearson's chi-squared or Fisher's exact test was used where appropriate. The level of significance was set at $p < 0.05$. The data management, statistical analysis, and computation of figures were conducted using R (R Development Core Team, Vienna, Austria, Version 4.1.1, 2021).

3. Results

3.1. Characteristics of the Study Population

From February 2020 to October 2020, 840 SARS-CoV-2-positive diagnosed patients were admitted to an ICU at a LEOSS study site (Table 1). The majority of the patients were between 46 and 85 years old (85.1%; 715/840), and 6.7% (56/840) were older than 85 years. A total of 602 of the 840 patients (71.7%) were male; the only age group without a male predominance was the 85+ age group. The most common comorbidities were hypertension (61.0%, 512/840), diabetes mellitus (28.1%; 236/840), chronic kidney disease (17.3%; 145/840), coronary artery disease (16.7%; 140/840), and atrial fibrillation (16.0%; 134/840). Only 13.9% of the patients (117/840) had no documented comorbidities; one comorbidity was documented for 22.0% of the patients (185/840), and multiple comorbidities (up to 14) were reported in 64.1% of the patients (538/840). Mechanical ventilation therapy was used in the vast majority of patients. In 21.5% of the patients (181/840), an attempt at non-invasive ventilation failed, requiring intubation; in 37.0% of the patients (311/840), intubation was performed without prior non-invasive ventilation. Exclusive non-invasive ventilation was documented in 10.4% of the patients (87/840). Extracorporeal membrane oxygenation (ECMO) was required in 13.6% of the patients (114/840). Still, 17.5% of the patients (147/840) did not receive mechanical ventilation therapy. The majority of the patients (66.2%, 556/840) had a length of stay in the ICU of 0–3 weeks; 264 of 840 patients (31.4%) received intensive care for 4–9 weeks, and for 2.4% of the patients (20/840), a length of treatment in the ICU exceeding 9 weeks was documented. The overall mortality rate was 46% (386/840).

Table 1. Epidemiological data of the total cohort, as well as subcohorts, subdivided according to the type of ventilation performed. ECMO: extracorporeal membrane oxygenation.

	Total Cohort	Subcohort: No Ventilation	Subcohort: Non-Invasive Ventilation	Subcohort: Invasive Ventilation	Subcohort: ECMO
Patient count	840	147	87	492	114
Age range (years)	<1 to >85	<1 to >85	36 to >85	9 to >85	26 to 85
Gender distribution (male/female)	602/238	92/55	60/27	357/135	93/21
Number of comorbidities	0 to 14	0 to 14	0 to 11	0 to 12	0 to 7
Length of stay in ICU (weeks)	0 to 10	0 to 10	0 to 6	0 to 10	0 to 10
Length of ventilation (weeks)	up to 9	-	up to 6	up to 9	up to 9
Mortality rate (%)	46.0	53.7	39.1	41.1	62.3

3.2. Community-Acquired Colonializations with Multidrug-Resistant Bacteria

Complete or at least partial information on colonializations with multidrug-resistant pathogens at baseline (say of positive SARS-CoV-2 diagnosis) was available for 71.2% of the patients (598/840). Among these, colonialization with 3MRGN was documented in 2.8% of the cases, with MRSA in 2.6% of the cases and VRE in 4.1% of the cases. However, the majority of the patients (75.1% of the cases) were declared free of colonialization with these bacteria on presentation. Information on 4MRGN was captured in the dataset, but so few infections were reported that details were not made available in the LEOSS Scientific Use File to maintain patient anonymity.

Examining in detail the patient subcohorts grouped by ventilation therapy performed (i.e., no ventilation, non-invasive ventilation, invasive ventilation, or ECMO) indicated no fundamental differences in colonialization prevalence with multidrug-resistant pathogens

(Figure 1). Thus, the data did not support the hypothesis that a community-acquired colonialization with a multidrug-resistant pathogen increased the risk of a critically ill COVID-19 patient to require invasive ventilation or ECMO therapy.

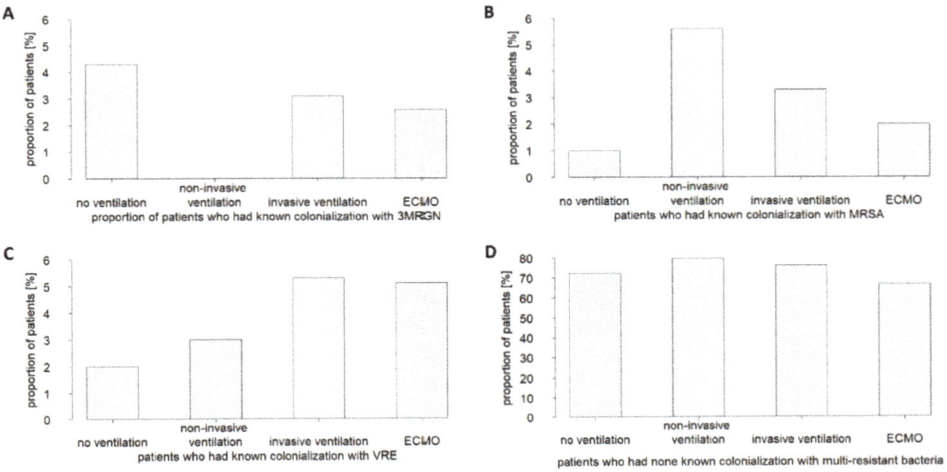

Figure 1. Prevalence of community-acquired colonializations with multidrug-resistant bacteria in patients critically ill with COVID-19 who received no ventilation therapy or were treated with non-invasive ventilation, invasive ventilation, or ECMO (extracorporeal membrane oxygenation). Shown are the proportions of patients who were colonized with (**A**) 3MRGN (multidrug-resistant Gram-negative bacteria), (**B**) MRSA (methicillin-resistant *Staphylococcus aureus*), or (**C**) VRE (vancomycin-resistant enterococci), or those where (**D**) no colonization was found.

Furthermore, the data demonstrated no association between a pre-existing colonialization with a multidrug-resistant bacterium and mortality in critically ill COVID-19 patients (Figure 2). No significant difference in colonialization status was observed between recovered and deceased patients (Figure 2).

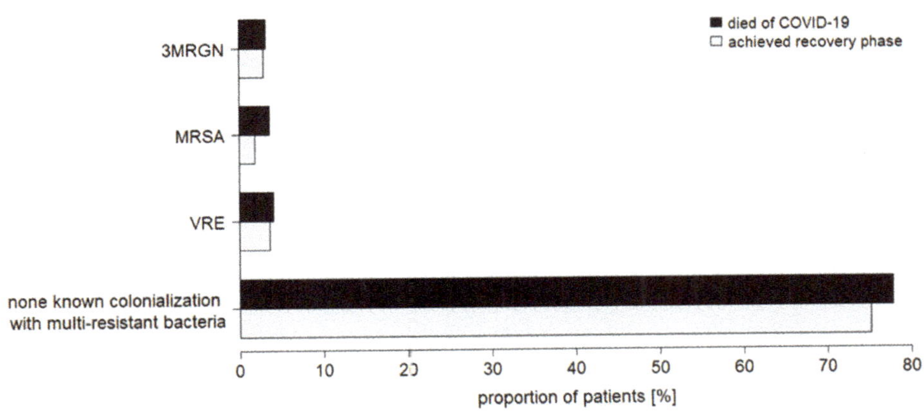

Figure 2. Prevalence of community-acquired colonializations with multidrug-resistant bacteria in recovered and deceased patients critically ill with COVID-19 (total cohort). MRGN: multidrug-resistant Gram-negative bacteria; MRSA: methicillin-resistant *Staphylococcus aureus*; VRE: vancomycin-resistant enterococci.

3.3. Healthcare-Associated Bacterial and Fungal Infections

Information on hospital-acquired bacterial and fungal infections of critically ill patients in the ICU was available for 806 cases (96.0% of the total cohort). Overall, secondary bacterial infection was documented for 326 patients in the critical phase (40.4% of the cases), and secondary fungal infection was documented for 118 patients in the critical phase (14.6% of the cases).

Remarkably, a comparative analysis of patient cohorts subdivided by ventilation therapy revealed significant differences in infection status (Figure 3). Healthcare-associated secondary infections with bacteria or fungi had an above-average prevalence in ECMO patients (bacterial co-infections in 60.5% of cases and fungal co-infections in 27.5% of cases). As such, ECMO patients were affected by nosocomial infections more frequently than invasively ventilated patients, in whom secondary co-infections with bacteria were documented in 43.1% of cases and with fungi in 15.4% of cases. However, a further lower, below-average prevalence of nosocomial infections was reported for the cohort of non-invasively ventilated patients (secondary bacterial co-infections in 23.0% of cases and secondary fungal co-infections in 6.9% of cases). In patients who did not receive ventilation, hospital-acquired bacterial co-infections were seen in 17.7% of cases and fungal co-infections in 0.9% of cases. These data support the hypothesis that invasive therapy procedures accompany an increased risk for healthcare-associated infections.

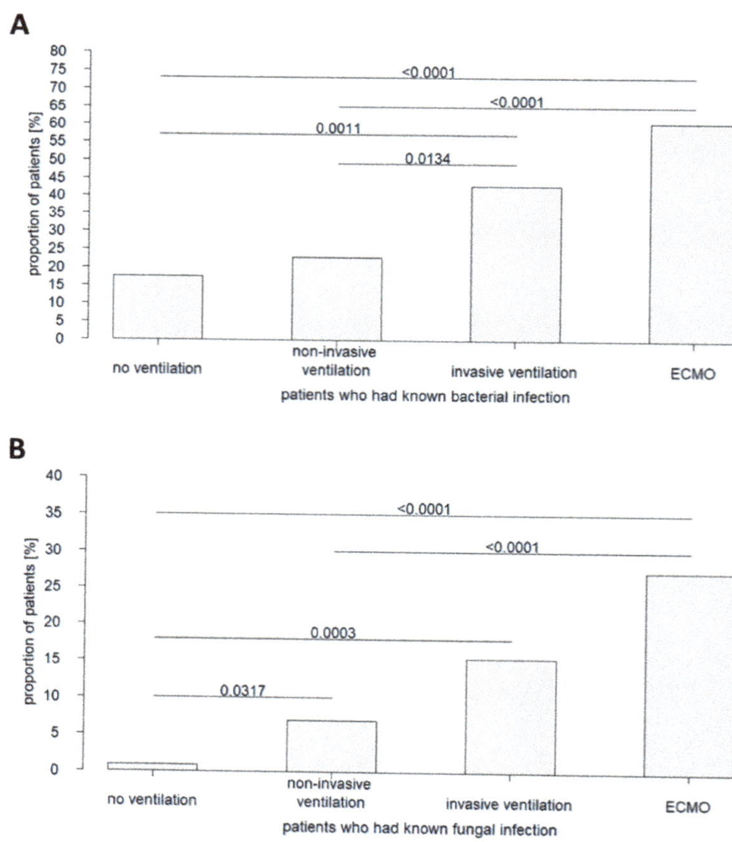

Figure 3. Prevalence of secondary infections in patients critically ill with COVID-19 who received no ventilation therapy or were treated with non-invasive ventilation, invasive ventilation, or ECMO. Shown are the proportions of patients with (**A**) bacterial and (**B**) fungal infections of nosocomial origin.

There were no significant differences in the frequencies of secondary bacterial or fungal infections when comparing critically ill COVID-19 patients who died or reached the recovery phase (Figure 4). Thus, no effect of hospital-acquired infections on outcome became apparent.

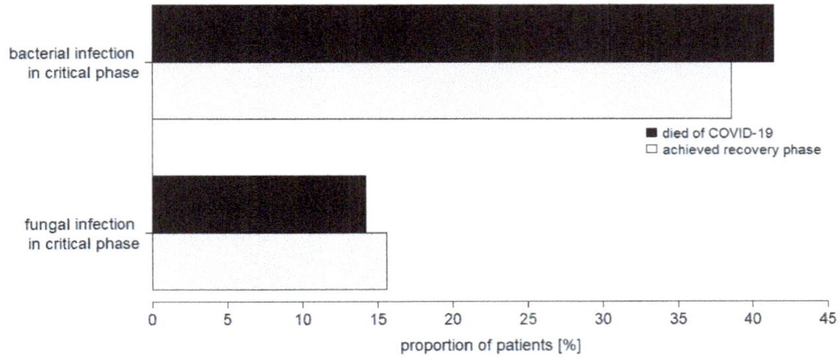

Figure 4. Prevalence of secondary bacterial and fungal infections in recovered and deceased patients critically ill with COVID-19 (total cohort).

3.4. Antimicrobial Therapy: Frequency of Use and Clinical Benefit

Antibiotic use data were available for only 285 critically ill patients with COVID-19 treated in the ICU (33.9% of the total cohort), an alarmingly low figure in terms of antimicrobial stewardship. An in-depth review of the pharmacologic treatment of these patients found that antibiotic treatment was the most frequently administered medication, even preceding epinephrine and sympathomimetics (Figure 5). Therefore, antibiotic therapy was administered in the vast majority of cases (88.4%), although bacterial infection was documented in just 40.4% of the overall patients and 47.6% of this particular patient subset.

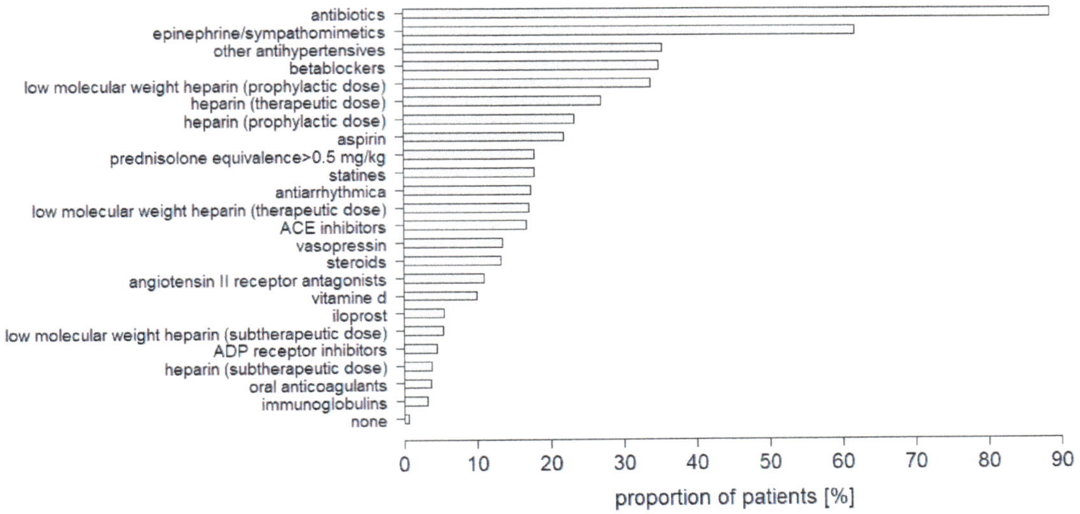

Figure 5. Medication used in intensive care for patients critically ill with COVID-19.

A detailed examination of the patient cohorts subdivided by ventilation therapy revealed that almost all the ECMO patients (95.7% of cases) received antibiotic treatment. In the case of invasive ventilation, antibiotics were administered in 91.8% of the patients. Substantially less frequently, but still at a high level, antibiotics were used in non-invasively ventilated patients (71.9% of cases) and patients who did not receive ventilation therapy (75.0% of cases).

There was no difference in antibiotic use frequency between patients who died as a result of COVID-19 infection and those who reached the recovery phase. However, considering the high rate of antibiotic use, especially in intubated patients and patients on ECMO therapy, no valid conclusion can be drawn from this as to the clinical benefit of antibiotic treatment. While empiric antibiotic treatment might prevent the development of nosocomial infections, it also impedes microbial pathogen detection and, therefore, hinders specific anti-infective therapy when needed.

4. Discussion

In the present study, the relations between the colonization with nosocomial bacteria, the rate of nosocomial infections, the necessity to undergo ventilation, and the mode of ventilation were examined for COVID-19 patients treated in an ICU. The results of the study showed that colonializations with 3MRGN, MRSA, and VRE were similar in non-ventilated patients and patients undergoing non-invasive, invasive, and oxygenation ventilation, indicating that colonization was not associated with ventilation or its invasiveness. Moreover, a colonization with multi-resistant bacteria was not associated with a fatal outcome. On the other hand, the number of nosocomial infections significantly correlated with the invasiveness of the ventilation modus, indicated by the finding that the lowest infection rates were observed in non-ventilated COVID-19 patients, while the highest numbers occurred in patients oxygenated with ECMO. However, these infections were not related with a fatal outcome.

Since the outbreak of the pandemic, the field of COVID-19 has evolved. Vaccines have been developed that are proven to reduce the need for ICU treatment in the case of a breakthrough infection [33]. Furthermore, there are now drug treatment strategies that, when initiated in a timely manner, can have a mitigating effect on disease severity and, thus, counteract the need for critical care [8]. However, a significant number of patients still develop respiratory insufficiency requiring admission to an ICU and targeted ventilation. The present study clearly demonstrated that such treatment was associated with an increased risk of secondary infections, with the invasiveness of the ventilation technique used being an influential variable. This is even more important as no correlation between patient characteristics, such as age or comorbidities, and the occurrence of secondary infections was found.

Infections pose a significant problem in ICUs [10,19,34–36], especially in patients with viral respiratory infections. In severe influenza, for example, bacterial co-infections have been described in up to 20% to 30% of cases, and superinfections have been associated with pronounced disease severity and a higher risk of death [17,26,28,29,34–36]. Consequently, in critically ill COVID-19 patients, the prevalence of bacterial and fungal co-infections, their impact on the clinical course, and appropriate antimicrobial therapy in a primarily viral disease are of particular importance.

Since the very beginning of the pandemic, co-infections of COVID-19 patients have been reported [18,19,35–39]. It needs to be noted that the several studies reporting superinfections have not distinctly distinguished between community-acquired and healthcare-associated infections, thus limiting the validity of these studies. Our study, however, clearly showed that the vast majority of patients had no evidence of colonialization with bacterial multidrug-resistant microorganisms at baseline, and only a single-digit percentage of patients was affected by colonialization with 3MRGN, MRSA, or VRE at hospital presentation. Thus, for the group of COVID-19 patients with a critical course, it resulted that colonization at the time of diagnosis of SARS-CoV-2 infection was rare, especially with regard to the most clinically relevant multidrug-resistant pathogens. Indeed, other studies have also reported low rates of early infection and, rather, direct the focus to nosocomial infection [17,34]. Reported rates of secondary bacterial infections in critically ill ICU patients with COVID-19 have ranged from 8.1% to 42.8% [13,17,18,34–39]. There is also a wide range of reported infection rates with respect to secondary fungal infections. As such, a meta-analysis of eight studies related to COVID-19 patients treated in an ICU setting reported an infection rate of 9.6% (95% CI 6.8–12.4) [37]. Specifically, in mechanically ventilated COVID-19 patients, a multicenter prospective cohort study found a rate of invasive fungal infections of 26.7% [40]. One can only speculate as to the causes of the wide range of case numbers reported. Workload, unfavorable physician- or nurse-to-patient ratios, and a lack of laboratory capacity, especially in the early months of the pandemic, might have partially limited the capability for widespread infection control. For additional consideration, especially for critically ill ICU patients, the true prevalence of secondary infections may be underestimated due to the untimely deaths of these patients. In any case, our study provided clear evidence that nosocomial infections of bacterial and fungal origin were common in COVID-19 patients receiving intensive care and warrant awareness and adequate management. There is a need for the proper diagnosis and effective treatment of not only bacterial but also fungal infections in COVID-19 patients receiving intensive care.

Critically ill COVID-19 patients undergo a variety of invasive interventions in the ICU, such as mechanical ventilation and catheterization, which promote bacterial and fungal infections [10,13,17,19,21,26,38,39,41] and are described to be more frequently subject to additive bacterial and fungal infections compared to patients treated in regular wards [13,35–39]. We were, therefore, interested in the impact of the level of therapeutic invasiveness on the prevalence of healthcare-associated infections. Indeed, our data clearly proved that non-ventilated ICU patients were at low risk for secondary infections. The risk of infection increased markedly, even when non-invasive ventilation was used. A dramatic rise in the proportion of patients with nosocomial infections was seen with the use of invasive ventilation, and even more so with ECMO therapy. Actually, in ECMO-treated patients, healthcare-associated bacterial infections were present in about two-thirds of cases and healthcare-associated fungal infections in nearly one-third of cases. Our data provided evidence that the techniques used in intensive care for the treatment of COVID-19-induced respiratory insufficiency differed significantly with respect to risk profiles for secondary infections. Based on these data, close infection control is recommended, especially when invasive methods are required.

There is ongoing discussion as to whether secondary infections impact mortality in COVID-19 patients. Some studies have reported an association of nosocomial infections with adverse outcome, whereas other studies have found no such correlation [19,20,37,39,41,42]. In our study, the rates of secondary infections of surviving and deceased COVID-19 patients were not significantly different. The same was true for community-acquired colonialization with 3MRGN, MRSA, and VRE. Patient-associated factors, such as pre-existing conditions, may be critical in determining whether co-infections ultimately impact survival. In a risk analysis, Silva et al. already showed that co-infections increased the risk of death, specifically in patients with obesity, cardiovascular disease, or diabetes mellitus [41]. Obesity, cardiovascular disease, and diabetes mellitus are known risk factors for a critical course of SARS-CoV-2 infection and are common in ICU patients (as in the present study cohort). This raises the possibility of a vicious circle. Large cohort studies are needed to investigate this in detail, with particular priority on ICU patients, given their high risk of developing secondary infections.

Several guidelines, such as those from the World Health Organization (WHO) and the Surviving Sepsis Campaign, advocate the use of empiric antibiotics in patients with severe COVID-19 [7,43]. This explains why, in our study, the absolute majority of patients (88.4%) were treated with antibiotics, despite the fact that only half of these patients had a positive finding of bacterial infection. Other studies have consistently reported hospitalized COVID-19 patients receiving antimicrobial therapy in 50% to 100% of cases [13,15,18,20,26,27,34,36,38]. The undifferentiated use of antimicrobial agents is known to increase selection pressure and may promote the spread of resistant bacterial strains. Indeed, there are concerns that the increased usage of antibiotics in the context of the COVID-19 pandemic may worsen the issue of multidrug-resistant pathogens worldwide [27–29,34]. Strict adherence to antibiotic stewardship programs, effective implementation of infection control procedures, and maintenance of established hygiene standards need to be upheld even in pandemic settings. This is particularly true for ICUs, as invasive treatments are key to the development of secondary infections, as illustrated by the present study.

Our study has certain limitations. Due to its retrospective nature, data availability was limited to the medical records added to the LEOSS registry. We did not have information of interest, such as the presence of antibiotic resistance or the type, dosage, and timing of antibiotic, antifungal, or immunosuppressant drugs. Accordingly, we could not make statements on these potential influencing factors. This study included ICU patients suffering from COVID-19 from Europe, predominantly Germany, which may limit the generalizability of our findings.

5. Conclusions

Healthcare-associated infections are common in critically ill COVID-19 patients treated in ICUs. Our study highlighted the importance of the type of intensive care treatment when it came to nosocomial infections. Patients receiving invasive ventilation had markedly increased rates of secondary bacterial and fungal infections compared with those receiving non-invasive treatment. Another distinct increase in infection rates was documented in ECMO-treated patients. This knowledge should inform future treatment decisions in the ICU.

Author Contributions: Conceptualization, S.B., D.E. and J.S.; methodology, S.B. and J.S.; validation, M.L.d.H., D.E. and J.S.; formal analysis, M.L.d.H. and J.S.; investigation, M.L.d.H., D.E. and J.S.; data curation, S.B., S.R., J.J.V., C.D.S., C.E.M.K., M.H., M.S. and F.H.; writing—original draft preparation, J.S.; writing—review and editing, M.L.d.H., S.B. and D.E.; visualization, M.L.d.H.; supervision, J.S.; project administration, J.S. All authors have read and agreed to the published version of the manuscript.

Funding: The LEOSS registry is supported by the German Center for Infection Research (DZIF) and the Willy Robert Pitzer Foundation.

Institutional Review Board Statement: The study was conducted in accordance with the Declaration of Helsinki. Approval for LEOSS was obtained from the applicable local ethics committees of all participating centers and registered at the German Clinical Trails Register (DRKS, No. S00021145).

Informed Consent Statement: Patient consent was waived, as the study was based on a Scientific Use File (SUF) generated from the Lean European Open Survey on SARS-CoV-2-Infected Patients (LEOSS) registry. For the LEOSS database, data collection was performed fully anonymized, only once per case, and retrospectively after treatment was finished or the patient had died.

Data Availability Statement: Patient data from the LEOSS registry are subject to the LEOSS governance, data use, and access policy (policy text available on https://leoss.net; accessed on 4 August 2022).

Acknowledgments: We express our deep gratitude to all the study teams supporting the LEOSS study. The LEOSS study group contributed at least 5 per million to the analyses of this study from: University Hospital Regensburg (Frank Hanses), University Hospital Freiburg (Siegbert Rieg), Technical University of Munich (Christoph Spinner), Hospital Ingolstadt (Stefan Borgmann), Klinikum Dortmund gGmbH, Hospital of University Witten/Herdecke (Martin Hower), University Hospital Frankfurt (Maria Vehreschild), University Hospital Wuerzburg (Nora Isberner), University Hospital Tuebingen (Siri Göpel), Hospital Maria Hilf GmbH Moenchengladbach (Juergen vom Dahl), University Hospital Augsburg (Christoph Roemmele), University Hospital Jena (Maria Madeleine Ruethrich), University Hospital Cologne (Norma Jung), University Hospital Erlangen (Richard Strauss), University Hospital Ulm (Beate Gruener), Hospital Bremen-Center (Christian Hohmann), Hospital Ernst von Bergmann (Lukas Tometten), Hospital Passau (Julia Lanznaster), University Hospital Saarland (Robert Bals), Municipal Hospital Karlsruhe (Christian Degenhardt), University Hospital Duesseldorf (Bjoern-Erik Jensen), University Hospital Heidelberg (Uta Merle), Johannes Wesling Hospital Minden Ruhr University Bochum (Kai Wille), University Hospital Dresden (Katja de With), Bundeswehr Hospital Koblenz (Dominic Rauschning), University Hospital of Giessen and

Marburg (Janina Trauth), University Hospital Essen (Sebastian Dolff), University Hospital Schleswig-Holstein Kiel (Anette Friedrichs), Elbland Hospital Riesa (Joerg Schubert), Malteser Hospital St. Franziskus Flensburg (Milena Milovanovic), Marien Hospital Herne Ruhr University Bochum (Timm Westhoff), Clinic Munich (Wolfgang Guggemos), Catholic Hospital Bochum (St. Josef Hospital) Ruhr University Bochum (Kerstin Hellwig), Practice for general medicine Drs. Elisabeth Schroedter & Gabriele Mueller-Joerger Kuenzelsau (Gabriele Mueller-Joerger), Hospital Universitari Arnau de Vilanova (Juan Antonio Schoenenberger-Arnaiz), Hospital Braunschweig (Jan Kielstein), Hospital Leverkusen (Lukas Eberwein), University Hospital Munich/ LMU (Michael von Bergwelt-Baildon), Agaplesion Diakonie Hospital Rotenburg (David Heigener), Thorax University Hospital Heidelberg (Felix Herth), and Evangelisches Hospital Saarbruecken (Mark Neufang). The LEOSS study infrastructure group includes: Jörg Janne Vehreschild (Goethe University Frankfurt), Susana M. Nunes de Miranda (University Hospital of Cologne), Carolin E. M. Koll (University Hospital of Cologne), Melanie Stecher (University Hospital of Cologne), Lisa Pilgram (Goethe University Frankfurt), Nick Schulze (University Hospital of Cologne), Sandra Fuhrmann (University Hospital of Cologne), Annika Claßen (University Hospital of Cologne), Bernd Franke (University Hospital of Cologne), and Fabian Praßer (Charité, Universitätsmedizin Berlin).

Conflicts of Interest: The authors declare no conflict of interest.

References

1. Sorbello, M.; El-Boghdadly, K.; Di Giacinto, I.; Cataldo, R.; Esposito, C.; Falcetta, S.; Merli, G.; Cortese, G.; Corso, R.M.; Bressan, F.; et al. The Italian coronavirus disease 2019 outbreak: Recommendations from clinical practice. *Anaesthesia* **2020**, *75*, 724–732. [CrossRef] [PubMed]
2. Bikdeli, B.; Madhavan, M.V.; Jimenez, D.; Chuich, T.; Dreyfus, I.; Driggin, E.; Der Nigoghossian, C.; Ageno, W.; Madjid, M.; Guo, Y.; et al. COVID-19 and Thrombotic or Thromboembolic Disease: Implications for Prevention, Antithrombotic Therapy, and Follow. *J. Am. Coll. Cardiol.* **2020**, *75*, 2950–2973. [CrossRef]
3. Pfeifer, M.; Ewig, S.; Voshaar, T.; Randerath, W.J.; Bauer, T.; Geiseler, J.; Dellweg, D.; Westhoff, M.; Windisch, W.; Schoenhofer, B.; et al. Position Paper for the State-of-the-Art Application of Respiratory Support in Patients with COVID-19. *Respiration* **2020**, *99*, 521–541. [CrossRef]
4. Kluge, S.; Janssens, U.; Welte, T.; Weber-Carstens, S.; Marx, G.; Karagiannidis, C. German recommendations for critically ill patients with COVID-19. *Med. Klin. Intensivmed.* **2020**, *115*, 111–114. [CrossRef]
5. Karagiannidis, C.; Mostert, C.; Hentschker, C.; Voshaar, T.; Malzahn, J.; Schillinger, G.; Klauber, J.; Janssens, U.; Marx, G.; Weber-Carstens, S.; et al. Case characteristics, resource use, and outcomes of 10 021 patients with COVID-19 admitted to 920 German hospitals: An observational study. *Lancet Resp. Med.* **2020**, *8*, 853–862. [CrossRef]
6. Thomas-Rueddel, D.; Winning, J.; Dickmann, P.; Ouart, D.; Kortgen, A.; Janssens, U.; Bauer, M. Coronavirus disease 2019 (COVID-19): Update for anesthesiologists and intensivists March 2020. *Anaesthesist* **2021**, *70*, 1–10. [CrossRef]
7. Alhazzani, W.; Moller, M.H.; Arabi, Y.M.; Loeb, M.; Gong, M.N.; Fan, E.; Oczkowski, S.; Levy, M.M.; Derde, L.; Dzierba, A.; et al. Surviving Sepsis Campaign: Guidelines on the management of critically ill adults with Coronavirus Disease 2019 (COVID-19). *Int. Care Med.* **2020**, *46*, 854–887. [CrossRef]
8. Fachgruppe COVRIIN beim Robert-Koch-Institut. Antivirale Therapie in der Frühphase einer SARS-CoV-2-Infektion: Bei Patienten mit Risikofaktoren für einen Schweren Verlauf von COVID-19 (bei Asymptomatischen Patienten oder Patienten mit milder COVID-19); Bewertung durch die Fachgruppe COVRIIN beim Robert Koch-Institut. Available online: https://www.rki.de/DE/Content/InfAZ/N/Neuartiges_Coronavirus/COVRIIN_Dok/Antivirale_Therapie_Fruehphase.pdf?__blob=publicationFile (accessed on 29 June 2022).
9. Fichtner, F.; Moerer, O.; Weber-Carstens, S.; Nothacker, M.; Kaisers, U.; Laudi, S.; Grp, G. Clinical Guideline for Treating Acute Respiratory Insufficiency with Invasive Ventilation and Extracorporeal Membrane Oxygenation: Evidence-Based Recommendations for Choosing Modes and Setting Parameters of Mechanical Ventilation. *Respiration* **2019**, *98*, 357–372. [CrossRef]
10. Vincent, J.L.; Bihari, D.J.; Suter, P.M.; Bruining, H.A.; White, J.; Nicolaschanoin, M.H.; Wolff, M.; Spencer, R.C.; Hemmer, M. The Prevalence of Nosocomial Infection in Intensive-Care Units in Europe—Results of the European Prevalence of Infection in Intensive-Care (EPIC) Study. *JAMA-J. Am. Med. Assoc.* **1995**, *274*, 639–644. [CrossRef]
11. Tobin, M.J. Basing Respiratory Management of COVID-19 on Physiological Principles. *Am. J. Respir. Crit. Care Med.* **2020**, *201*, 1319–1320. [CrossRef]
12. Chiurlo, M.; Mastrangelo, A.; Ripa, M.; Scarpellini, P. Invasive fungal infections in patients with COVID-19: A review on pathogenesis, epidemiology, clinical features, treatment, and outcomes. *New Microbiol.* **2021**, *44*, 71–83. [PubMed]
13. Chong, W.H.; Saha, B.K.; Ramani, A.; Chopra, A. State-of-the-art review of secondary pulmonary infections in patients with COVID-19 pneumonia. *Infection* **2021**, *49*, 591–605. [CrossRef] [PubMed]

14. Russell, C.D.; Fairfield, C.J.; Drake, T.M.; Turtle, L.; Seaton, R.A.; Wootton, D.G.; Sigfrid, L.; Harrison, E.M.; Docherty, A.B.; de Silva, T.I.; et al. Co-infections, secondary infections, and antimicrobial use in patients hospitalised with COVID-19 during the first pandemic wave from the ISARIC WHO CCP-UK study: A multicentre, prospective cohort study. *Lancet Microbe* **2021**, *2*, E354–E365. [CrossRef] [PubMed]
15. Rawson, T.M.; Moore, L.S.P.; Zhu, N.; Ranganathan, N.; Skolimowska, K.; Gilchrist, M.; Satta, G.; Cooke, G.; Holmes, A. Bacterial and Fungal Coinfection in Individuals With Coronavirus: A Rapid Review To Support COVID-19 Antimicrobial Prescribing. *Clin. Infect. Dis.* **2020**, *71*, 2459–2468. [CrossRef] [PubMed]
16. Manna, S.; Baindara, P.; Mandal, S.M. Molecular pathogenesis of secondary bacterial infection associated to viral infections including SARS-CoV-2. *J. Infect. Public Health* **2020**, *13*, 1397–1404. [CrossRef]
17. Pasero, D.; Cossu, A.P.; Terragni, P. Multi-Drug Resistance Bacterial Infections in Critically Ill Patients Admitted with COVID-19. *Microorganisms* **2021**, *9*, 1773. [CrossRef]
18. Fehér, Á.; Szarvas, Z.; Lehoczki, A.; Fekete, M.; Fazekas-Pongor, V. Co-infections in COVID-19 patients and correlation with mortality rate. Minireview. *Physiol. Int.* **2022**, *109*, 1–8. [CrossRef]
19. Roudbary, M.; Kumar, S.; Kumar, A.; Cernakova, L.; Nikoomanesh, F.; Rodrigues, C.F. Overview on the Prevalence of Fungal Infections, Immune Response, and Microbiome Role in COVID-19 Patients. *J. Fungi* **2021**, *7*, 720. [CrossRef]
20. Grasselli, G.; Scaravilli, V.; Mangioni, D.; Scudeller, L.; Alagna, L.; Bartoletti, M.; Bellani, G.; Biagioni, E.; Bonfanti, P.; Bottino, N.; et al. Hospital-Acquired Infections in Critically Ill Patients With COVID-19. *Chest* **2021**, *160*, 454–465. [CrossRef]
21. Falcone, M.; Tiseo, G.; Giordano, C.; Leonildi, A.; Menichini, M.; Vecchione, A.; Pistello, M.; Guarracino, F.; Ghiadoni, L.; Forfori, F.; et al. Predictors of hospital-acquired bacterial and fungal superinfections in COVID-19: A prospective observational study. *J. Antimicrob. Chemother.* **2021**, *76*, 1078–1084. [CrossRef]
22. Klein, E.Y.; Monteforte, B.; Gupta, A.; Jiang, W.; May, L.; Hsieh, Y.-H.; Dugas, A. The frequency of influenza and bacterial coinfection: A systematic review and meta-analysis. *Influenza Other Respir. Viruses* **2016**, *10*, 394–403. [CrossRef] [PubMed]
23. MacIntyre, C.R.; Chughtai, A.A.; Barnes, M.; Ridda, I.; Seale, H.; Toms, R.; Heywood, A. The role of pneumonia and secondary bacterial infection in fatal and serious outcomes of pandemic influenza a(H1N1)pdm09. *BMC Infect. Dis.* **2018**, *18*, 637. [CrossRef]
24. Rice, T.W.; Rubinson, L.; Uyeki, T.M.; Vaughn, F.L.; John, B.B.; Miller, R.R., II; Higgs, E.; Randolph, A.G.; Smoot, B.E.; Thompson, B.T.; et al. Critical illness from 2009 pandemic influenza A virus and bacterial coinfection in the United States. *Crit. Care Med.* **2012**, *40*, 1487–1498. [CrossRef] [PubMed]
25. Esper, F.P.; Spahlinger, T.; Zhou, L. Rate and influence of respiratory virus co-infection on pandemic (H1N1) influenza disease. *J. Infect.* **2011**, *63*, 260–266. [CrossRef]
26. Cox, M.J.; Loman, N.; Bogaert, D.; O'Grady, J. Co-infections: Potentially lethal and unexplored in COVID-19. *Lancet Microbe* **2020**, *1*, E11. [CrossRef]
27. Getahun, H.; Smith, I.; Trivedi, K.; Paulin, S.; Balkhy, H.H. Tackling antimicrobial resistance in the COVID-19 pandemic. *Bull World Health Organ.* **2020**, *98*, 442. [CrossRef]
28. Ginsburg, A.S.; Klugman, K.P. COVID-19 pneumonia and the appropriate use of antibiotics. *Lancet Glob. Health* **2020**, *8*, E1453–E1454. [CrossRef]
29. Huttner, B.D.; Catho, G.; Pano-Pardo, J.R.; Pulcini, C.; Schouten, J. COVID-19: Don't neglect antimicrobial stewardship principles! *Clin. Microbiol. Infect.* **2020**, *26*, 808–810. [CrossRef]
30. Meintrup, D.; Borgmann, S.; Seidl, K.; Stecher, M.; Jakob, C.E.M.; Pilgram, L.; Spinner, C.D.; Rieg, S.; Isberner, N.; Hower, M.; et al. Specific Risk Factors for Fatal Outcome in Critically Ill COVID-19 Patients: Results from a European Multicenter Study. *J. Clin. Med.* **2021**, *10*, 3855. [CrossRef]
31. Jakob, C.E.M.; Kohlmayer, F.; Meurers, T.; Vehreschild, J.J.; Prasser, F. Design and evaluation of a data anonymization pipeline to promote Open Science on COVID-19. *Sci. Data* **2020**, *7*, 435. [CrossRef]
32. Jakob, C.E.M.; Borgmann, S.; Duygu, F.; Behrends, U.; Hower, M.; Merle, U.; Friedrichs, A.; Tometten, L.; Hanses, F.; Jung, N.; et al. First results of the Lean European Open Survey on SARS-CoV-2-Infected Patients (LEOSS). *Infection* **2021**, *49*, 63–73. [CrossRef] [PubMed]
33. Bahl, A.; Johnson, S.; Maine, G.; Garcia, M.H.; Nimmagadda, S.; Qu, L.; Chen, N.-W. Vaccination reduces need for emergency care in breakthrough COVID-19 infections: A multicenter cohort study. *Lancet Reg Health Am.* **2021**, *4*, 100065. [CrossRef] [PubMed]
34. Peghin, M.; Vena, A.; Graziano, E.; Giacobbe, D.R.; Tascini, C.; Bassetti, M. Improving management and antimicrobial stewardship for bacterial and fungal infections in hospitalized patients with COVID-19. *Ther. Adv. Infect. Dis.* **2022**, *9*, 28. [CrossRef]
35. Lansbury, L.; Lim, B.; Baskaran, V.; Lim, W.S. Co-infections in people with COVID-19: A systematic review and meta-analysis. *J. Infect.* **2020**, *81*, 266–275. [CrossRef] [PubMed]
36. Langford, B.J.; So, M.; Raybardhan, S.; Leung, V.; Westwood, D.; MacFadden, D.R.; Soucy, J.-P.R.; Daneman, N. Bacterial co-infection and secondary infection in patients with COVID-19: A living rapid review and meta-analysis. *Clin. Microbiol. Infect.* **2020**, *26*, 1622–1629. [CrossRef] [PubMed]
37. Alhumaid, S.; Al Mutair, A.; Al Alawi, Z.; Alshawi, A.M.; Alomran, S.A.; Almuhanna, M.S.; Almuslim, A.A.; Bu Shafia, A.H.; Alotaibi, A.M.; Ahmed, G.Y.; et al. Coinfections with Bacteria, Fungi, and Respiratory Viruses in Patients with SARS-CoV-2: A Systematic Review and Meta-Analysis. *Pathogens* **2021**, *10*, 809. [CrossRef]

38. Langford, B.J.; So, M.; Leung, V.; Raybardhan, S.; Lo, J.; Kan, T.; Leung, F.; Westwood, D.; Daneman, N.; MacFadden, D.R.; et al. Predictors and microbiology of respiratory and bloodstream bacterial infection in patients with COVID-19: Living rapid review update and meta-regression. *Clin. Microbiol. Infect.* **2022**, *28*, 491–501. [CrossRef]
39. Musuuza, J.S.; Watson, L.; Parmasad, V.; Putman-Buehler, N.; Christensen, L.; Safdar, N. Prevalence and outcomes of co-infection and superinfection with SARS-CoV-2 and other pathogens: A systematic review and meta-analysis. *PLoS ONE* **2021**, *16*, e0251170. [CrossRef]
40. White, P.L.; Dhillon, R.; Cordey, A.; Hughes, H.; Faggian, F.; Soni, S.; Pandey, M.; Whitaker, H.; May, A.; Morgan, M.; et al. A national strategy to diagnose COVID-19 associated invasive fungal disease in the ICU. *Clin. Infect. Dis.* **2020**, *73*, e1634–e1644. [CrossRef]
41. Silva, D.L.; Lima, C.M.; Magalhaes, V.C.R.; Baltazar, L.M.; Peres, N.T.A.; Caligiorne, R.B.; Moura, A.S.; Fereguetti, T.; Martins, J.C.; Rabelo, L.F.; et al. Fungal and bacterial coinfections increase mortality of severely ill COVID-19 patients. *J. Hosp. Infect.* **2021**, *113*, 145–154. [CrossRef]
42. Bardi, T.; Pintado, V.; Gomez-Rojo, M.; Escudero-Sanchez, R.; Azzam Lopez, A.; Diez-Remesal, Y.; Martinez Castro, N.; Ruiz-Garbajosa, P.; Pestana, D. Nosocomial infections associated to COVID-19 in the intensive care unit: Clinical characteristics and outcome. *Europ. J. Clin. Microbiol. Infect. Dis.* **2021**, *40*, 495–502. [CrossRef] [PubMed]
43. Wolrd Health Organization. Living Guidance for Clinical Management of COVID-19: Living Guidance, 23 November 2021. Available online: https://apps.who.int/iris/bitstream/handle/10665/349321/WHO-2019-nCoV-clinical-2021.2-eng.pdf (accessed on 4 August 2022).

Journal of
Clinical Medicine

MDPI

Article

The Burden of Carbapenem-Resistant *Acinetobacter baumannii* in ICU COVID-19 Patients: A Regional Experience

Giorgia Montrucchio [1,2,*,†], Silvia Corcione [3,4,†], Tommaso Lupia [3], Nour Shbaklo [3], Carlo Olivieri [5], Miriam Poggioli [5], Aline Pagni [6], Davide Colombo [6], Agostino Roasio [7], Stefano Bosso [7], Fabrizio Racca [8], Valeria Bonato [8], Francesco Della Corte [9], Stefania Guido [9], Andrea Della Selva [10], Enrico Ravera [10], Nicoletta Barzaghi [11], Martina Cerrano [11], Pietro Caironi [12], Giacomo Berta [12], Cecilia Casalini [13], Bruno Scapino [13], Michele Grio [14], Massimiliano Parlanti Garbero [14], Gabriella Buono [15], Federico Finessi [15], Simona Erbetta [16], Paola Federica Sciacca [16], Gilberto Fiore [16], Alessandro Cerutti [16], Sergio Livigni [17], Daniela Silengo [17], Fulvio Agostini [18], Maurizio Berardino [18], Mauro Navarra [19], Silvia Vendramin [19], Enzo Castenetto [20], Marco Maria Liccardi [20], Emilpaolo Manno [21], Luca Brazzi [1,2] and Francesco Giuseppe De Rosa [3]

1 Department of Surgical Sciences, University of Turin, 10126 Turin, Italy
2 Department of Anaesthesia, Critical Care and Emergency—Città Della Salute e Della Scienza Hospital, Corso Dogliotti 14, 10126 Turin, Italy
3 Department of Medical Sciences, Infectious Diseases, University of Turin, 10126 Turin, Italy
4 Division of Geographic Medicine, Tufts University School of Medicine, Boston, MA 02111, USA
5 S.C. Anestesia e Rianimazione, Ospedale Sant'Andrea, 13100 Vercelli, Italy
6 S.C. Anestesia e Rianimazione, Ospedale SS. Trinità—Borgomanero—ASL NO, 28021 Borgomanero, Italy
7 S.C. Anestesia e Rianimazione, Ospedale Cardinal Massaia, 14100 Asti, Italy
8 S.C. Anestesia e Rianimazione, Ospedale SS. Arrigo e Biagio, 15121 Alessandria, Italy
9 Department of Translational Medicine, Maggiore della Carità Hospital, University of Eastern Piedmont—UPO, 28100 Novara, Italy
10 S.C. Anestesia e Rianimazione, ASL CN2, 12060 Verduno, Italy
11 Dipartimento di Emergenza ed Aree Critiche, SSD Rianimazione, A.S.O.S. Croce e Carle, 12100 Cuneo, Italy
12 S.C.DU Anestesia e Rianimazione, AOU S. Luigi Gonzaga, Dipartimento di Oncologia, Università degli Studi di Torino, 10043 Orbassano, Italy
13 S.C. Anestesia e Rianimazione, Ospedale di Ivrea, ASL TO4, 10015 Ivrea, Italy
14 S.C. Anestesia e Rianimazione, Ospedale di Rivoli, 10098 Rivoli, Italy
15 S.C. Rianimazione Generale, AO Ordine Mauriziano, 10128 Turin, Italy
16 S.C. Anestesia e Rianimazione Moncalieri-Carmagnola, ASL TO5, 10023 Chieri, Italy
17 S.C Anestesia e Rianimazione Ospedale S. Giovanni Bosco, ASL Città di Torino, 10144 Turin, Italy
18 S.C. Anestesia e Rianimazione, Presidio CTO, AOU Città della Salute e della Scienza, 10126 Turin, Italy
19 S.C. Anestesia e Rianimazione, Ospedale Martini, ASL Città di Torino, 10149 Turin, Italy
20 S.C. Anestesia e Rianimazione, Ospedale di Chivasso, ASL TO4, 10034 Chivasso, Italy
21 S.C. Anestesia e Rianimazione, Ospedale Maria Vittoria, ASL Città di Torino, 10144 Turin, Italy
* Correspondence: giorgiagiuseppina.montrucchio@unito.it
† These authors contributed equally to this work.

Citation: Montrucchio, G.; Corcione, S.; Lupia, T.; Shbaklo, N.; Olivieri, C.; Poggioli, M.; Pagni, A.; Colombo, D.; Roasio, A.; Bosso, S.; et al. The Burden of Carbapenem-Resistant *Acinetobacter baumannii* in ICU COVID-19 Patients: A Regional Experience. *J. Clin. Med.* **2022**, *11*, 5208. https://doi.org/10.3390/jcm11175208

Academic Editor: Daniel L. Herr

Received: 11 July 2022
Accepted: 26 August 2022
Published: 2 September 2022

Abstract: Since the beginning of the COVID-19 pandemic, the impact of superinfections in intensive care units (ICUs) has progressively increased, especially carbapenem-resistant *Acinetobacter baumannii* (CR-Ab). This observational, multicenter, retrospective study was designed to investigate the characteristics of COVID-19 ICU patients developing CR-Ab colonization/infection during an ICU stay and evaluate mortality risk factors in a regional ICU network. A total of 913 COVID-19 patients were admitted to the participating ICUs; 19% became positive for CR-Ab, either colonization or infection (n = 176). The ICU mortality rate in CR-Ab patients was 64.7%. On average, patients developed colonization or infection within 10 ± 8.4 days from ICU admission. Scores of SAPS II and SOFA were significantly higher in the deceased patients (43.8 ± 13.5, p = 0.006 and 9.5 ± 3.6, $p < 0.001$, respectively). The mortality rate was significantly higher in patients with extracorporeal membrane oxygenation (12; 7%, p = 0.03), septic shock (61; 35%, $p < 0.001$), and in elders (66 ± 10, $p < 0.001$). Among the 176 patients, 129 (73%) had invasive infection with CR-Ab: 105 (60.7%) Ventilator-Associated Pneumonia (VAP), and 46 (26.6%) Bloodstream Infections (BSIs). In 22 cases (6.5%), VAP was associated with concomitant BSI. Colonization was reported in 165 patients (93.7%). Mortality was significantly higher in patients with VAP (p = 0.009). Colonized patients who did not develop invasive infections had a higher survival rate ($p < 0.001$). Being colonized by CR-Ab was associated with a higher risk of developing invasive infections ($p < 0.001$). In a multivariate analysis, risk factors significantly associated with mortality were age (OR = 1.070; 95% CI (1.028–1.115) $p = 0.001$) and CR-Ab colonization (OR = 5.463 IC95% 1.572–18.988, $p = 0.008$). Constant infection-control measures are necessary to stop the spread of *A. baumannii* in the hospital environment especially at this time of the SARS-CoV-2 pandemic, with active surveillance cultures and the efficient performance of a multidisciplinary team.

Keywords: *Acinetobacter baumannii; Acinetobacter* infections; intensive care unit; COVID-19; SARS-CoV-2, nosocomial infections; carbapenems; multidrug resistance; antimicrobial drug resistance; critical care

1. Introduction

The Gram-negative aerobic bacillus *Acinetobacter baumannii (A. baumannii)* primarily causes hospital-acquired infections in especially fragile patients with prolonged hospitalization and with long-term exposition to broad-spectrum antibiotic treatment. It is characterized by disinfection resistance, and its high pathogenicity is increased by the production of a polysaccharide capsule and by the ability to form biofilms [1]. Furthermore, due to the acquisition of multiple antimicrobial resistance, especially to carbapenems, it has been recognized as a major public health concern [2] and considered as "priority 1" (critical) in the World Health Organization (WHO)'s first list of "priority pathogens" resistant to antibiotics, including the 12 families of bacteria most dangerous for human health and for which new antimicrobials are urgently required [3].

It is well known that *A. baumannii* exhibits a wide variety of mechanisms of resistance to antibiotic agents, as differential clones had been isolated in Europe [4]. *A. baumannii* includes several mechanisms of resistance such as lipopolysaccharide expression disorders, permeability alterations due to porins, and the production of active efflux pumps. In particular, resistance to carbapenems is related to numerous beta-lactamases with carbapenemase activity, including type OXA carbapenemases—both constitutive or acquired. Moreover, a transmissible resistance mechanism of colistin, called mobile colistin resistance (MCR), was discovered. Up to ten families with MCR and more than 100 variants of Gram-negative bacteria have been reported worldwide. Even though few have been reported from *Acinetobacter* spp. and *Pseudomonas* spp., it is important to closely monitor the epidemiology of MCR genes in these pathogens [1,4].

A. baumannii can survive for long periods on surfaces, including human skin and dry surfaces (up to 33 days) [5], and this ability might facilitate its persistence in intensive care units (ICUs), rightly considered as the epicenters of carbapenem-resistant *A. baumannii* (CR-Ab) infections [6,7]. Some specific factors may increase the potential of cross-transmission: the heavy colonization of the patient, the colonization of the surfaces surrounding the patients, and the total number of patients colonized in the unit at the same time [8]. CR-Ab also has a further important feature, namely its tendency to generate outbreaks, generally transmitted through the hands of healthcare workers, contaminated equipment, and the healthcare environment [7,9,10].

The most frequently reported risk factors for CR-Ab infections are prior colonization, the severity of illness, the need for mechanical ventilation (particularly in case of prolonged duration), immunosuppression, malignancies, chronic pulmonary diseases, respiratory failure on admission, previous antimicrobial therapy, previous sepsis in ICU, previous use of carbapenems and third generation cephalosporins, long ICU stay [11], and a consequent greater degree of exposure to infected or colonized patients in the hospital environment [12,13].

Overall, CR-Ab is accountable for more than 12% of the cases of hospital-acquired bloodstream infections (BSI) in the ICU, with wide geographic variations: it is frequent in Southern Europe, Middle Eastern countries, Asia, and South America, whereas it is rare in Northern European countries and Australia [14]. CR-Ab is a common cause of ICU-acquired pneumonia, particularly late-onset pneumonia [15].

Since the beginning of the COVID-19 pandemic, the impact of superinfections in ICU patients has progressively increased and many studies have shown that the rate of BSIs [16] and Ventilator-Associated Pneumonia (VAP) [17] is raised compared to that observed in non-COVID-19 patients [18–21]. It has also been reported that the prevalence of Gram-negative multi-drug resistant organisms, especially *A. baumannii*, known to increase mortality, seems to have escalated [22,23].

In Italy, various experiences of multidrug-resistant (MDR) bacterial infection in COVID-19 and its impact on patient outcomes have been published, [24] but few describe specifically *A. baumannii* cases. Several studies showed that MDR infection arose after a median time of 8 [4–11] days and the incidence rate ratio of MDR infection in ICU increased in the COVID-19 period [25,26].

Despite the above evidence and the interest in superinfections from multidrug-resistant pathogens, particularly CR-Ab in ICU patients with COVID-19 [27], to date, no multicenter study has been conducted with the aim of better describing the phenomenon.

The present multicenter retrospective study was designed to investigate the characteristics of COVID-19 ICU patients who developed CR-Ab colonization or infection during their ICU stay and evaluate risk factors for ICU mortality in a regional ICU network.

2. Materials and Methods

2.1. Study Design and Population

This was an observational, multicenter, and retrospective study. Nineteen COVID-19 ICUs in the Piedmont Region, Italy, were invited to participate in an observational, multicenter, retrospective study to describe the incidence of colonization and infection with CR-Ab in SARS-CoV2 pneumonia patients admitted to ICUs between 1 July and 31 December 2021.

The data sources were the hospital administrative records and the Microbiology Laboratory database. Data acquisition and analysis were performed in accordance with the protocols approved by the local Ethics Committee (Ethics Committee: Comitato Etico Interaziendale A.O.U. Città della Salute e della Scienza di Torino—A.O. Ordine Mauriziano—A.S.L. Città di Torino; ethics approval number 0031285). Written informed consent was waived according to Italian regulations due to the retrospective nature of this study. The study was conducted according to the guidelines of the Declaration of Helsinki.

All consecutive adult (≥18 years) patients admitted to the ICU and presenting CR-Ab colonization or infection during the study period were enrolled. All patients were followed up until the hospital discharge to compute: ICU, 28-day and overall mortality, length of ICU and hospital stay.

2.2. Context

During the study period, several infection control programs were active in the ICUs involved, with specific leadership and scope. Surveillance cultures (tracheal aspirate, rectal swab, urinary culture) were performed weekly; universal screening for carbapenem-producing *Enterobacterales* (CPE) and *A. baumannii* using rectal swabs was performed upon admission to the ICU and then once a week. In mechanically ventilated patients, the surveillance of respiratory samples (tracheal aspirates or bronchoalveolar lavage) was also performed at least once a week, with some differences between the different centers. Blood cultures or bronchoalveolar lavage cultures were performed on clinical decision.

2.3. Definitions

Pneumonia by Severe Acute Respiratory Syndrome Coronavirus 2 (SARS-CoV-2) was defined based on real-time polymerase chain reaction (RT-PCR) on at least one low respiratory tract specimen [28].

The occurrence of colonization and/or infection with *A. baumannii* was assessed from the date of ICU admission to ICU discharge. It was considered only once at the time of the first incidence of a positive sample. Colonization was defined as bacterial isolation without clinical signs or symptoms suggestive of infection. Infection was defined according to the Centers for Disease Control and Prevention (CDC) criteria [29]. Carbapenem resistance was defined according to the EUCAST criteria [30].

All episodes of VAP and/or BSI, as well as the development of septic shock with the requirement of vasoactive drugs [31], were registered according to the European Centre for Disease Prevention and Control (ECDC) current definitions [32].

2.4. Microbiology

A. baumannii and CPE strains from blood, respiratory, and rectal samples were collected in accordance with active surveillance screening and following local guidelines. Rectal swabs were collected from hospitalized patients and screened for CPE by combining culture-based detection and the identification of carbapenemase type.

We identified CR-Ab according to the European Committee on Antimicrobial Susceptibility Testing (EUCAST) criteria of carbapenem resistance. Cultures were analyzed with the BD BACTECTM FX system (Becton Dickinson) according to EUCAST breakpoint tables. The identification of microorganisms was conducted with mass spectrometry MALDI-TOF (Matrix-Assisted Laser Desorption Ionization Time-of-Flight) and VITEK®, whereas susceptibility to antibiotic molecules was tested using VITEK 2 (VITEK® according to EUCAST breakpoint tables). The whole-genome sequencing of CR-Ab isolates collected from blood cultures and respiratory samples was not available in the pandemic context. The clonal relationship of CR-Ab isolates was currently not investigated.

2.5. Statistical Analysis

Data were entered and analyzed using SPSS version 27. Statistical significance was defined as less than 0.05. Descriptive analysis was reported as frequencies, percentages, means, and standard deviations. Categorical variables, demographics, and clinical characteristics were compared against mortality using the Chi-squared test. Continuous variables were tested for normality by the Kolmogorov–Smirnov test. Non-normally distributed variables were evaluated using the Mann–Whitney test.

Significant values in the univariate analysis were evaluated with a multivariate model: a logistic regression model for mortality to assess independent predictors. The odds ratio was reported with corresponding 95% confidence intervals.

3. Results

Sixteen ICUs joined the data collection. Four of them had no cases of CR-Ab in COVID-19 patients. The first data collection was completed in May 2021. The review of the data by independent investigators was completed in the months of June–September 2021.

During the study period, 913 COVID-19 patients were admitted to the participating ICUs. Of them, 19% became positive for CR-Ab, either colonization or infection ($n = 176$). The ICU mortality rate in patients with *A. baumannii* was as high as 64.7% ($n = 112$) (Table 1).

Table 1. Demographic and general characteristics of COVID-19 ICU patients with CR-Ab.

Variable (*n*; %)	**Total** 176 (100%)	**Survived** 61 (35.3%)	**Dead** 112 (64.7%)	***p*-Value**
Demographics				
Males	136 (78.6)	48 (67.6%)	88 (78.6%)	0.986
Age	65.35 ± 10.3	62.84 ± 10.7	66.44 ± 10	**<0.001**
BMI	30.8 ± 7.3	31.33 ± 7.4	30.83 ± 7.36	0.858
Ex-smoker	8 (4.5)	4 (6.5)	4 (3.5)	0.372
Smoker	8 (4.5)	3 (4.9)	5 (4.5)	0.892
Obese	52 (29.5)	20 (32.8)	32 (28.6)	0.563

Table 1. *Cont.*

Variable (*n*; %)	Total 176 (100%)	Survived 61 (35.3%)	Dead 112 (64.7%)	*p*-Value
Comorbidities				
Cardiovascular disease	118 (67)	38 (62.3)	80 (71.4)	0.218
Diabetes	39 (22.1)	12 (19.7)	27 (24.1)	0.505
Hematologic disease	2 (1.1)	1 (1.6)	1 (0.9)	0.661
Chronic pulmonary disease	22 (12.5)	6 (9.8)	16 (14.3)	0.401
Renal failure	15 (8.5)	5 (8.1)	10 (8.9)	0.870
Active neoplasm	7 (4)	2 (3.3)	5 (4.5)	0.705
Autoimmune disease	18 (10.2)	6 (9.8)	12 (10.7)	0.857
Immunodepression	4 (2.3)	2 (3.3)	2 (1.8)	0.532
Clinical characteristics				
ICU length of stay	24.27 ± 17.9	25.7 ± 20.58	24.1 ± 18.22	0.930
Days to infection/colonization from hospital admission	17.31 ± 13.3	17.2 ± 13.44	17.31 ± 12.34	0.718
Days to infection/colonization from ICU admission	10.69 ± 8.4	10.63 ± 8.38	10.69 ± 8.42	0.585
Referral	54 (30.7)	17 (27.9)	37 (33)	0.483
ECMO	13 (7.4)	1 (1.6)	12 (10.7)	**0.031**
SAPS II	42.28 ± 13.37	41.6 ± 13	43.88 ± 13.5	**0.006**
SOFA	8.3 ± 3.7	6 ± 2.6	9.5 ± 3.6	**<0.001**
ARDS on admission	165 (93.2)	59 (96.7)	106 (94.6)	0.534
Septic shock	67 (38.1)	6 (9.8)	61 (54.5)	**<0.001**
Colistin sensitive	159 (90.3)	53 (86.9)	106 (94.6)	0.074
Colistin resistant	14 (7.9)	8 (13.1)	6 (5.3)	
Carbapenem-resistant	122 (69.3)	46 (75.4)	76 (67.8)	0.479
Invasive infections				
CR-Ab VAP	105 (59.6)	29 (47.5)	76 (67.8)	**0.009**
CR-Ab BSI	46 (41.1)	14 (22.9)	32 (28.6)	0.424
CR-Ab + **co-infection**				
K. pneumoniae—KPC	29 (16.5)	11 (18)	18 (16.1)	0.726
MRSA	8 (4.5)	3 (4.9)	5 (4.5)	0.892
VRE	7 (4)	3 (4.9)	4 (3.6)	0.668
Enteric pathogens	55 (31.2)	18 (29.5)	37 (33)	0.634
Colonization				
CR-Ab	165 (93.7)	58 (95)	104 (92.8)	0.567
Cp-*K.pneumoniae*	14 (7.9)	4 (6.5)	10 (8.9)	0.585
VRE	1 (0.6)	1 (1.6)	0	0.174
E.coli	2 (1.1)	2 (3.2)	0	0.054
Candida spp	8 (4.5)	3 (4.9)	5 (4.5)	0.892
MRSA	5 (2.8)	1 (1.6)	4 (3.6)	0.469
Other	74 (42)	28 (45.9)	46 (41.1)	0.587
Combination treatment with colistin				
Total colistin treatment	100 (56.8)	33 (54)	67 (59.8)	0.466
Colistin monotherapy	10 (5.7)	1 (1.6)	9 (8)	0.085
Meropenem	37 (21)	16 (26.2)	21 (18.7)	0.252
Ampicillin sulbactam	32 (18.1)	9 (14.7)	23 (20.5)	0.349
Rifampicin	30 (17)	9 (14.7)	21 (18.7)	0.507
Tigecycline	15 (8.5)	2 (3.2)	13 (11.6)	0.063
Vancomycin	7 (4)	3 (4.9)	4 (3.6)	0.668
Ceftazidime-avibactam	7 (4)	1 (1.6)	6 (5.3)	0.236
Only colonized/infected vs. mortality				
CR-Ab colonized (without infection)	47 (26.7)	25 (40.9)	22 (19.6)	**<0.001**
CR-Ab infected (without colonization)	11 (6.2)	3 (4.9)	8 (7.1)	0.567

List of abbreviations: intensive care unit, ICU; carbapenem-resistant *Acinetobacter baumannii*, CR-Ab; number, *n*; Body Mass Index, BMI; extracorporeal membrane oxygenation, ECMO; Simplified Acute Physiology Score, SAPS; Sequential Organ Failure Assessment, SOFA; Acute Respiratory Distress Syndrome, ARDS; Ventilator-Associated Pneumonia, VAP; Bloodstream infection, BSI; *K.pneumoniae* producing KPC; methicillin-resistant *Staphylococcus aureus*, MRSA; vancomycin-resistant *Enterococcus*, VRE. bold was used for $p < 0.05$.

The majority of patients were males (136; 78.6%), with a median age of 65 ± 10.3 years. The average Simplified Acute Physiology Score (SAPS) II and Sequential Organ Failure Assessment (SOFA) scores were 42 ± 13.37 and 8.3 ± 3.7, respectively. Leading comorbidities were cardiovascular diseases (118 patients, 67%), obesity (52 patients, 29.5%), diabetes (39 patient, 22.1%), and chronic pulmonary disease (22 patients, 12.5%) Around 31% of patients were transferred from one hospital to another; 93.2% of them presented acute respiratory distress syndrome upon ICU admission. The mean length of stay in the ICU was 24 ± 18 days. On average, patients developed colonization or infection within 10 ± 8.4 days from ICU admission.

The scores of SAPS II and SOFA were significantly higher in the deceased patients (43.8 ± 13.5, $p = 0.006$ and 9.5 ± 3.6, $p < 0.001$, respectively). Furthermore, the mortality rate was significantly higher in patients with extracorporeal membrane oxygenation (ECMO; 12; 7%, $p = 0.03$), septic shock (61; 35%, $p < 0.001$), and in elders (66 ± 10, $p < 0.001$) (Table 1).

Among the 176 patients enrolled in the study, 129 (73%) had invasive infection with CR-Ab, distributed as follows: 105 (60.7%) VAP and 46 (26.6%) BSI. In 22 cases (6.5%), VAP was associated with concomitant BSI. Colonization was reported in 165 patients (93.7%). Of note, 118 patients previously colonized by CR-Ab developed invasive infections, while 11 patients developed infection without any known previous colonization. Mortality was significantly higher in patients with VAP ($p = 0.009$). Colonized patients who did not develop invasive infections had a higher survival rate ($p < 0.001$; Table 1). Being colonized by CR-Ab was associated with a higher risk of developing invasive infections ($p < 0.001$).

Co-infections with carbapenem-resistant Klebsiella pneumoniae and enteric pathogens were seen in 29 (17%) and 55 (32%) patients, respectively.

Most of the CR-Ab isolates (159, 90.3%) were sensitive to colistin. Colistin was used to treat the majority (100, 56.8%) of the patients. Most commonly, it was administered with meropenem, ampicillin-sulbactam, and rifampicin (21%, 18.1%, and 17%), respectively. However, no difference in mortality rate was observed between different therapies.

In the multivariate analysis (Table 2), risk factors that were significantly associated with mortality were age (OR = 1.070; 95% CI (1.028–1.115) $p = 0.001$) and CR-Ab colonization (OR = 5.463 ic 96% 1.572–18.988 $p = 0.008$).

Table 2. Multivariate analysis for mortality.

Variables	p Value	OR	95% C.I.for EXP(B)	
			Lower	Upper
Age	0.001	**1.070**	1.028	1.115
SAPS II	0.145	1.022	0.992	1.053
VAP	0.451	1.568	0.487	5.049
CR-Abcolonization	0.008	**5.463**	1.572	18.988

List of abbreviations: Simplified Acute Physiology Score, SAPS; Ventilator-Associated Pneumonia, VAP; carbapenem-resistant *Acinetobacter baumannii*, CR-Ab. bold was used for $p < 0.05$.

4. Discussion

Bacterial and fungal superinfections represent a severity factor with a high impact on the morbidity and mortality of critically ill patients with COVID-19 [33,34]. This aspect is even more essential in countries burdened by a high rate of multidrug-resistant bacteria, such as Italy [35], where an increasing number of CR-Ab infections have been seen in the last years.

In the present multicentric study, conducted on 16 ICUs in the Piedmont region during the COVID-19 pandemic, it was found that 19% of ICU COVID-19 patients became positive for CR-Ab, either colonization or infection, during an ICU stay. Although the whole-genome sequencing of CR-Ab isolates was not available in the pandemic context and the clonal relationship of CR-Ab isolates was currently not investigated, this elevated percentage and some epidemiological factors deserve very high attention. Furthermore, the mortality rate in patients with CR-Ab was as high as 64.7%, significantly higher than the overall mortality in critically ill COVID-19 patients [36].

To the best of our knowledge, this is the first multicenter regional study reporting the impact of CR-Ab colonization and severe infection in ICUs during the COVID-19 pandemic. Interestingly, our analysis refers to the so-called Italian "second-wave" of the pandemic, when the global emergency scenario of the first months of the pandemic had extensively changed. A recent multicenter, cross-sectional study compared the rates of colonization and infection with carbapenemase-producing *Enterobacterales* (CPE) and/or CR-Ab in two study periods, pre and during the COVID-19 pandemic. No significant change in either incidence rate ratios and weekly trends in CPE colonization and infection was observed, while the incidence rate ratios of colonization and infection with CR-Ab increased by 7.5- and 5.5-fold, respectively, during the COVID-19 period. A clonal lineage was demonstrated and appointed for the occurrence of horizontal transmission [26].

Other authors previously highlighted that, during the first wave of the COVID-19 pandemic, several factors could have favored the emergence and spread of antimicrobial-resistant bacteria in hospitals [25], such as the overload of hospitalized patients, especially in intensive care, favoring patient-to-patient transmission [37]; the initial overuse of antibiotics for suspected bacterial co/super-infections [38]; the possible delay in providing microbiological culture and sensitivities results due to the COVID-19 overload [39]. During the first months of the pandemic, in several countries, including Italy, a lack of appropriate protective personal equipment and health personnel hired on an emergency basis to respond to the COVID-19 pandemic, sometimes impeding adequate training in infection prevention and control, were common. However, that may not be completely true in the period of our study, when the first pandemic phase with its need for reorganization was already over.

Other factors may have contributed to the described spread of CR-Ab infections.

First of all, the need for the referral of critically ill patients (e.g., requiring ECMO [40]) and the high number of patients transferred from one hospital to another may have facilitated the dissemination of cases at the regional level. Even the structural characteristics of ICUs (new, re-opened, or already functioning before the COVID-19 pandemic) may also have played a role, in terms of spaces dedicated to patients and workstations, devices, and hospital pathways between departments (e.g., emergency department, radiology). In fact, CR-Ab cross-transmission between equipment (ventilators, infusion pumps, hemodialysis machines, ultrasound devices) and COVID-19 patients may also partly explain the onset of this outbreak.

Focusing on the identification and characterization of Enterococcus faecium, Staphylococcus aureus, Klebsiella pneumoniae, *Acinetobacter baumannii*, Pseudomonas aeruginosa, and Enterobacter spp. (ESKAPE) bacteria and their possible clonal spread in medical devices, patients, and medical personnel in the ICU, a recent work [41] has shown that 91% of the analyzed sites were colonized by bacteria (pathogenic and commensal), where *S. aureus* and *A. baumannii* MDR showed a high incidence, and *A. baumannii* MDR showed a clonal distribution in surfaces, patients, and health personnel.

It is in fact known that even when there is the scrupulous protection of medical personnel to avoid the transmission of SARS-CoV-2 from patients to health personnel, the transmission of other pathogens such as ESKAPE bacteria is not automatically avoided. In a previous study in ICUs, it was shown that the bacterial recontamination of contact surfaces occurred after 4 h after standard cleaning with detergents with chlorine-releasing agents, isopropyl alcohol, and sodium hypochlorite [42]. Moreover, COVID-19 critically ill patients often require prolonged hospitalizations, and it is known that staying in an intensive care setting for a long time—as well as immunosuppression, the need for prolonged previous antibiotic therapies, and the invasiveness of care—are known risk factors for infections with multidrug-resistant pathogens.

In our analysis, the median ICU length of stay was high (24.27 ± 17.9 days), with a time lag before the development of colonization or the onset of invasive infection of 17.31 ± 13.3 days of hospital stay and 10.69 ± 8.4 days of ICU stay, respectively.

Some other factors must be taken into account in the analyzed population. Certainly, patient severity had an impact on mortality, with statistical significance for the need for ECMO support, higher SAPS and SOFA scores, and the presence of septic shock as infection presentation. Similar to other settings, the use of steroids might be related to a higher risk of developing MDR infection [43]. Concerning the impact of VAP in CR-Ab infected patients, the diagnosis of VAP may have been made difficult by the presence of the radiological and clinical signs of COVID-19 pneumonia, which made it even more difficult to apply the classical criteria and the consequent definition of VAP.

The presence of colonization preceding the infection represented, in our series, a risk factor with respect to mortality. It is well known from the literature that colonization does not require any "pre-emptive" therapy if the patient has no clinical signs of infection, but these data confirmed the finding that colonization remains one of the main risk factors for invasive infections and represent a "wake up call" regarding the frailty of our patients. Therefore, implementing an early pre-emptive therapy in cases of known colonization, at the time of clinical worsening, is one of the main steps to improve survival in this setting.

As previously reported in the literature, the role of combination therapy is widely debated in the absence of definitive evidence [44,45]. The data are insufficient for a more completed analysis, but the unmet need for new and effective therapies is of paramount importance considering the mortality of these critically ill patients.

The presence of multi-bacterial co-infections is a further interesting fact, able to describe not only the fragility of the patients but also the delicate hospital ecology and to reinforce the need for effective and strict control measures. In particular, the combination of various Gram-negative pathogens describes the context of our ICUs and may be the consequence of the high use of empiric broad-spectrum antibiotic therapies used in COVID patients not only at home but also in the early stages of hospitalization.

Our study has several limitations. First, the retrospective nature of the study and therapeutic management on the risk of *A. baumannii* infection. Secondly, the lack of data on the total number of COVID-19 ICU patients did not allow a comparison of risk factors and outcomes. Third, as the clonal relationship was not investigated, it is impossible to define the common origin of the burden of infections or a relationship, at least in the high number of referral patients. Moreover, it was not possible to obtain a cumulative antibiogram for antibiotic classes to show the overall sensibility of different strains. Finally, the local epidemiology and the need to re-organize the capacity, spaces, and staff of our ICUs during the pandemic could limit the generalizability of our results.

5. Conclusions

The need to not neglect antimicrobial stewardship principles during the COVID-19 pandemic has already been recently underlined [46], as well as the importance of enhancing infection control activities directed against antimicrobial resistance. In continuity with this message, our study remarks on the need to pursue antimicrobial stewardship principles during the COVID-19 pandemic, and infection control activities targeted against the spread of antimicrobial resistance inside and between hospitals.

During a pandemic, not only in the first phases, but especially later in the time course, infection control activities should be revised and eventually re-modulated according to the new organizational structures. Constant infection-control measures are necessary to stop the spread of *A. baumannii* in the hospital environment, prevent outbreaks, and lower mortality rates, especially at this time of the SARS-CoV-2 pandemic. Stricter barrier measures need to be implemented, increasing the effectiveness of screening and surveillance for *A. baumannii*, especially when resistant to carbapenems. The active surveillance culture and efficient performance of a multidisciplinary team will be highly important in detecting and controlling the CR-Ab outbreak in COVID-19 ICUs.

Author Contributions: Conceptualization, G.M., S.C., L.B. and F.G.D.R.; Data curation, G.M., T.L., N.S., C.O., M.P., A.P., D.C., A.R., S.B., F.R., V.B., F.D.C., S.G., A.D.S., E.R., N.B., M.C., P.C., G.B. (Giacomo Berta), C.C., B.S., M.G., M.P.G., G.B. (Gabriella Buono), F.F., S.E., P.F.S., G.F., A.C., S.L., D.S., F.A., M.B., M.N., S.V., E.C., M.M.L. and E.M.; Formal analysis, G.M., S.C., T.L., N.S. and F.G.D.R.; Investigation, G.M., S.C., T.L., C.O., M.P., A.P., D.C., A.R., S.B., F.R., V.B., F.D.C., S.G., A.D.S., E.R., N.B., M.C., P.C., G.B. (Giacomo Berta), C.C., B.S., M.G., M.P.G., G.B. (Gabriella Buono), F.F., S.E., P.F.S., G.F., A.C., S.L., D.S., F.A., M.B., M.N., S.V., E.C., M.M.L. and E.M.; Methodology, G.M., S.C., L.B. and F.G.D.R.; Project administration, L.B. and F.G.D.R.; Resources, L.B. and F.G.D.R.; Software, N.S.; Supervision, G.M., P.C., L.B. and F.G.D.R.; Validation, S.C. and P.C.; Writing—original draft, G.M., S.C., M.C. and M.G.; Writing—review & editing, T.L., N.S., C.O., M.P., A.P., D.C., A.R., S.B., F.R., V.B., F.D.C., S.G., A.D.S., E.R., N.B., P.C., G.B. (Giacomo Berta), C.C., B.S., M.P.G., G.B. (Gabriella Buono), F.F., S.E., P.F.S., G.F., A.C., S.L., D.S., F.A., M.B., M.N., S.V., E.C., M.M.L., E.M., L.B. and F.G.D.R. All authors have read and agreed to the published version of the manuscript.

Funding: This research received no external funding.

Institutional Review Board Statement: Data acquisition and analysis were performed in accordance with the protocols approved by the local Ethics Committee (Ethics Committee: Comitato Etico Interaziendale A.O.U. Città della Salute e della Scienza di Torino—A.O. Ordine Mauriziano—A.S.L. Città di Torino; ethics approval number 0031285). The study was conducted according to the guidelines of the Declaration of Helsinki.

Informed Consent Statement: Written informed consent was waived according to Italian regulations due to the retrospective nature of this study.

Data Availability Statement: The datasets used and analyzed during the current network meta-analysis are available from the corresponding author upon reasonable request.

Acknowledgments: We would thank all the study collaborators in each ICU involved, and in particular: Rosario Urbino, Città della Salute e della Scienza Hospital, Torino; Marinella Zanierato, Città Della Salute e Della Scienza Hospital, Torino; Ilaria De Benedetto, Department of Medical Sciences, Infectious Diseases, University of Turin; Alessandro Bianchi, Ospedale Cardinal Massaia, Asti; Silvio Borrè, AO S.Andrea, Vercelli; Lucio Boglione, University of Eastern Piedmont, Italy; Serena Querio, Maggiore della Carità Hospital, Novara; Arianna Abascià, AO Ordine Mauriziano Torino; Valerio Del Bono, AO Santa Croce e Carle, Cuneo; Guido Chichino, AO SS. Arrigo e Biagio, Alessandria; and Chiara Scaletti, Ospedale di Rivoli, Italy.

Conflicts of Interest: The authors declare no conflict of interest regarding this manuscript.

References

1. Garnacho-Montero, J.; Timsit, J.F. Managing Acinetobacter baumannii infections. *Curr. Opin. Infect. Dis.* **2019**, *32*, 69–76. [CrossRef] [PubMed]
2. Cassini, A.; Högberg, L.D.; Plachouras, D.; Quattrocchi, A.; Hoxha, A.; Simonsen, G.S.; Colomb-Cotinat, M.; Kretzschmar, M.E.; Devleesschauwer, B.; Cecchini, M.; et al. Attributable deaths and disability-adjusted life-years caused by infections with antibiotic-resistant bacteria in the EU and the European Economic Area in 2015: A population-level modelling analysis. *Lancet Infect. Dis.* **2019**, *19*, 56–66. [CrossRef]
3. Tacconelli, E.; Carrara, E.; Savoldi, A.; Harbarth, S.; Mendelson, M.; Monnet, D.L.; Pulcini, C.; Kahlmeter, G.; Kluytmans, J.; Carmeli, Y.; et al. WHO Pathogens Priority List Working Group. Discovery, research, and development of new antibiotics: The WHO priority list of antibiotic-resistant bacteria and tuberculosis. *Lancet Infect. Dis.* **2018**, *18*, 318–327. [CrossRef]
4. Fitzpatrick, M.A.; Ozer, E.A.; Hauser, A.R. Utility of Whole-Genome Sequencing in Characterizing Acinetobacter Epidemiology and Analyzing Hospital Outbreaks. *J. Clin. Microbiol.* **2016**, *54*, 593–612. [CrossRef]
5. Howard, A.; O'Donoghue, M.; Feeney, A.; Sleator, R.D. Acinetobacter baumannii: An emerging opportunistic pathogen. *Virulence* **2012**, *3*, 243–250. [CrossRef]
6. Jawad, A.; Seifert, H.; Snelling, A.M.; Heritage, J.; Hawkey, P.M. Survival of Acinetobacter baumannii on dry surfaces: Comparison of outbreak and sporadic isolates. *J. Clin. Microbiol.* **1998**, *36*, 1938–1941. [CrossRef]
7. Meschiari, M.; Lòpez-Lozano, J.M.; Di Pilato, V.; Gimenez-Esparza, C.; Vecchi, E.; Bacca, E.; Orlando, G.; Franceschini, E.; Sarti, M.; Pecorari, M.; et al. A five-component infection control bundle to permanently eliminate a carbapenem-resistant *Acinetobacter baumannii* spreading in an intensive care unit. *Antimicrob. Resist. Infect. Control.* **2021**, *10*, 123. [CrossRef] [PubMed]
8. Masse, J.; Elkalioubie, A.; Blazejewski, C.; Ledoux, G.; Wallet, F.; Poissy, J.; Preau, S.; Nseir, S. Colonization pressure as a risk factor of ICU-acquired multidrug resistant bacteria: A prospective observational study. *Eur. J. Clin. Microbiol. Infect. Dis.* **2017**, *36*, 797–805. [CrossRef]

9. Munoz-Price, L.S.; Arheart, K.; Nordmann, P.; Boulanger, A.E.; Cleary, T.; Alvarez, R.; Pizano, L.; Namias, N.; Kett, D.H.; Poirel L. Eighteen years of experience with Acinetobacter baumannii in a tertiary care hospital. *Crit. Care Med.* **2013**, *41*, 2733–2742 [CrossRef]
10. Escudero, D.; Cofiño, L.; Forcelledo, L.; Quindós, B.; Calleja, C.; Martín, L. Control of an Acinetobacter baumannii multidrug resistance endemic in the ICU. Recalling the obvious. *Med. Intensiv.* **2017**, *41*, 497–499. [CrossRef]
11. Garnacho-Montero, J.; Dimopoulos, G.; Poulakou, G.; Akova, M.; Cisneros, J.M.; De Waele, J.; Petrosillo, N.; Seifert, H.; Timsit, J.F.; Vila, J.; et al. Task force on management and prevention of Acinetobacter baumannii infections in the ICU. *Intensive Care Med.* **2015**, *41*, 2057–2075. [CrossRef] [PubMed]
12. Lee, H.Y.; Chen, C.L.; Wu, S.R.; Huang, C.W.; Chiu, C.H. Risk factors and outcome analysis of Acinetobacter baumannii complex bacteremia in critical patients. *Crit. Care Med.* **2014**, *42*, 1081–1088. [CrossRef] [PubMed]
13. Huang, H.; Chen, B.; Liu, G.; Ran, J.; Lian, X.; Huang, X.; Wang, N.; Huang, Z. A multi-center study on the risk factors of infection caused by multi-drug resistant Acinetobacter baumannii. *BMC Infect. Dis.* **2018**, *18*, 11. [CrossRef] [PubMed]
14. Tabah, A.; Koulenti, D.; Laupland, K.; Misset, B.; Valles, J.; Bruzzi de Carvalho, F.; Paiva, J.A.; Cakar, N.; Ma, X.; Eggimann, P.; et al. Characteristics and determinants of outcome of hospital-acquired bloodstream infections in intensive care units: The EUROBACT International Cohort Study. *Intensive Care Med.* **2012**, *38*, 1930–1945. [CrossRef]
15. Koulenti, D.; Tsigou, E.; Rello, J. Nosocomial pneumonia in 27 ICUs in Europe: Perspectives from the EU-VAP/CAP study. *Eur. J. Clin. Microbiol. Infect. Dis.* **2017**, *36*, 1999–2006. [CrossRef]
16. Ripa, M.; Galli, L.; Poli, A.; Oltolini, C.; Spagnuolo, V.; Mastrangelo, A.; Muccini, C.; Monti, G.; De Luca, G.; Landoni, G.; et al. COVID-BioB study group. Secondary infections in patients hospitalized with COVID-19: Incidence and predictive factors. *Clin. Microbiol. Infect.* **2021**, *27*, 451–457. [CrossRef]
17. Giacobbe, D.R.; Battaglini, D.; Enrile, E.M.; Dentone, C.; Vena, A.; Robba, C.; Ball, L.; Bartoletti, M.; Coloretti, I.; Di Bella, S.; et al. Incidence and Prognosis of Ventilator-Associated Pneumonia in Critically Ill Patients with COVID-19: A Multicenter Study. *J. Clin. Med.* **2021**, *10*, 555. [CrossRef]
18. Sharifipour, E.; Shams, S.; Esmkhani, M.; Khodadadi, J.; Fotouhi-Ardakani, R.; Koohpaei, A.; Doosti, Z.; Ej Golzari, S. Evaluation of bacterial co-infections of the respiratory tract in COVID-19 patients admitted to ICU. *BMC Infect. Dis.* **2020**, *20*, 646. [CrossRef]
19. Gottesman, T.; Fedorowsky, R.; Yerushalmi, R.; Lellouche, J.; Nutman, A. An outbreak of carbapenem-resistant *Acinetobacter baumannii* in a COVID-19 dedicated hospital. *Infect. Prev. Pract.* **2021**, *3*, 100113. [CrossRef]
20. Shinohara, D.R.; Dos Santos Saalfeld, S.M.; Martinez, H.V.; Altafini, D.D.; Costa, B.B.; Fedrigo, N.H.; Tognim, M.C.B. Outbreak of endemic carbapenem-resistant *Acinetobacter baumannii* in a coronavirus disease 2019 (COVID-19)-specific intensive care unit. *Infect. Control. Hosp. Epidemiol.* **2021**, *43*, 815–817. [CrossRef]
21. Nasir, N.; Rehman, F.; Omair, S.F. Risk factors for bacterial infections in patients with moderate to severe COVID-19: A case-control study. *J. Med. Virol.* **2021**, *93*, 4564–4569. [CrossRef] [PubMed]
22. Bardi, T.; Pintado, V.; Gomez-Rojo, M.; Escudero-Sanchez, R.; Azzam Lopez, A.; Diez-Remesal, Y.; Martinez Castro, N.; Ruiz-Garbajosa, P.; Pestaña, D. Nosocomial infections associated to COVID-19 in the intensive care unit: Clinical characteristics and outcome. *Eur. J. Clin. Microbiol. Infect. Dis.* **2021**, *40*, 495–502. [CrossRef] [PubMed]
23. Liu, Y.; Wang, Q.; Zhao, C.; Chen, H.; Li, H.; Wang, H.; CARES Network. Prospective multi-center evaluation on risk factors, clinical characteristics and outcomes due to carbapenem resistance in *Acinetobacter baumannii* complex bacteraemia: Experience from the Chinese Antimicrobial Resistance Surveillance of Nosocomial Infections (CARES) Network. *J. Med. Microbiol.* **2020**, *69*, 949–959. [PubMed]
24. Montrucchio, G.; Corcione, S.; Sales, G.; Curtoni, A.; De Rosa, F.G.; Brazzi, L. Carbapenem-resistant Klebsiella pneumoniae in ICU-admitted COVID-19 patients: Keep an eye on the ball. *J. Glob. Antimicrob. Resist.* **2020**, *23*, 398–400. [CrossRef] [PubMed]
25. Karruli, A.; Boccia, F.; Gagliardi, M.; Patauner, F.; Ursi, M.P.; Sommese, P.; De Rosa, R.; Murino, P.; Ruocco, G.; Corcione, A.; et al. Multidrug-Resistant Infections and Outcome of Critically Ill Patients with Coronavirus Disease 2019: A Single Center Experience. *Microb. Drug Resist.* **2021**, *27*, 1167–1175. [CrossRef]
26. Pascale, R.; Bussini, L.; Gaibani, P.; Bovo, F.; Fornaro, G.; Lombardo, D.; Ambretti, S.; Pensalfine, G.; Appolloni, L.; Bartoletti, M.; et al. Carbapenem-resistant bacteria in an intensive care unit during the coronavirus disease 2019 (COVID-19) pandemic: A multicenter before-and-after cross-sectional study. *Infect. Control. Hosp. Epidemiol.* **2021**, *43*, 461–466. [CrossRef]
27. Rangel, K.; Chagas, T.P.G.; De-Simone, S.G. *Acinetobacter baumannii* Infections in Times of COVID-19 Pandemic. *Pathogens* **2021**, *10*, 1006. [CrossRef]
28. World Health Organization. Laboratory Testing for 2019 Novel Coronavirus (2019-nCoV) in Suspected Human Cases. Available online: https://www.who.int/publications-detail/laboratory-testing-strategy-recommendations-for-covid-19-interim-guidance (accessed on 10 July 2022).
29. Horan, T.C.; Andrus, M.; Dudeck, M.A. CDC/NHSN surveillance definition of health care-associated infection and criteria for specific types of infections in the acute care setting. *Am. J. Infect. Control.* **2008**, *36*, 309–332. [CrossRef]
30. EUCAST. Breakpoint Tables for Interpretation of MICs and Zone Diameters. Version 11.0. 2020. Available online: http://www.eucast.org/clinical_breakpoints/ (accessed on 10 July 2022).
31. Singer, M.; Deutschman, C.S.; Seymour, C.W.; Shankar-Hari, M.; Annane, D.; Bauer, M.; Bellomo, R.; Bernard, G.R.; Chiche, J.D.; Coopersmith, C.M.; et al. The Third International Consensus Definitions for Sepsis and Septic Shock (Sepsis-3). *JAMA* **2016**, *315*, 801–810. [CrossRef]

32. Plachouras, D.; Lepape, A.; Suetens, C. ECDC definitions and methods for the surveillance of healthcare-associated infections in intensive care units. *Intensive Care Med.* **2018**, *44*, 2216–2218. Erratum in *Intensive Care Med.* **2018**, *44*, 2020. [CrossRef]
33. Grasselli, G.; Cattaneo, E.; Florio, G. Secondary infections in critically ill patients with COVID-19. *Crit. Care* **2021**, *25*, 317. [CrossRef] [PubMed]
34. Montrucchio, G.; Lupia, T.; Lombardo, D.; Stroffolini, G.; Corcione, S.; De Rosa, F.G.; Brazzi, L. Risk factors for invasive aspergillosis in ICU patients with COVID-19: Current insights and new key elements. *Ann. Intensive Care* **2021**, *11*, 136. [CrossRef] [PubMed]
35. European Centre for Disease Prevention and Control (ECDC) ECDC. Surveillance of Antimicrobial Resistance in Europe 2018. 2019. Available online: https://www.ecdc.europa.eu/en/publications-data/surveillance-antimicrobial-resistance-europe-2018 (accessed on 10 July 2022).
36. Oliveira, E.; Parikh, A.; Lopez-Ruiz, A.; Carrilo, M.; Goldberg, J.; Cearras, M.; Fernainy, K.; Andersen, S.; Mercado, L.; Guan, J.; et al. ICU outcomes and survival in patients with severe COVID-19 in the largest health care system in central Florida. *PLoS ONE* **2021**, *16*, e0249038. [CrossRef] [PubMed]
37. Grasselli, G.; Pesenti, A.; Cecconi, M. Critical Care Utilization for the COVID-19 Outbreak in Lombardy, Italy: Early Experience and Forecast During an Emergency Response. *JAMA* **2020**, *323*, 1545–1546. [CrossRef]
38. Langford, B.J.; So, M.; Raybardhan, S.; Leung, V.; Westwood, D.; MacFadden, D.R.; Soucy, J.R.; Daneman, N. Bacterial co-infection and secondary infection in patients with COVID-19: A living rapid review and meta-analysis. *Clin. Microbiol. Infect.* **2020**, *26*, 1622–1629. [CrossRef]
39. Vaughn, V.M.; Gandhi, T.N.; Petty, L.A.; Patel, P.K.; Prescott, H.C.; Malani, A.N.; Ratz, D.; McLaughlin, E.; Chopra, V.; Flanders, S.A. Empiric Antibacterial Therapy and Community-onset Bacterial Coinfection in Patients Hospitalized with Coronavirus Disease 2019 (COVID-19): A Multi-hospital Cohort Study. *Clin. Infect. Dis.* **2021**, *72*, e533–e541. [CrossRef]
40. Montrucchio, G.; Sales, G.; Urbino, R.; Simonetti, U.; Bonetto, C.; Cura Stura, E.; Simonato, E.; Fuoco, G.; Fanelli, V.; Brazzi, L. ECMO Support and Operator Safety in the Context of COVID-19 Outbreak: A Regional Center Experience. *Membranes* **2021**, *11*, 334. [CrossRef]
41. Durán-Manuel, E.M.; Cruz-Cruz, C.; Ibáñez-Cervantes, G.; Bravata-Alcantará, J.C.; Sosa-Hernández, O.; Delgado-Balbuena, L.; León-García, G.; Cortés-Ortíz, I.A.; Cureño-Díaz, M.A.; Castro-Escarpulli, G.; et al. Clonal dispersion of Acinetobacter baumannii in an intensive care unit designed to patients COVID-19. *J. Infect. Dev. Ctries.* **2021**, *15*, 58–68. [CrossRef]
42. Wilson, A.P.; Smyth, D.; Moore, G.; Singleton, J.; Jackson, R.; Gant, V.; Jeanes, A.; Shaw, S.; James, E.; Cooper, B.; et al. The impact of enhanced cleaning within the intensive care unit on contamination of the near-patient environment with hospital pathogens: A randomized crossover study in critical care units in two hospitals. *Crit. Care Med.* **2011**, *39*, 651–658. [CrossRef]
43. Fanelli, V.; Montrucchio, G.; Sales, G.; Simonetti, U.; Bonetto, C.; Rumbolo, F.; Mengozzi, G.; Urbino, R.; Pizzi, C.; Richiardi, L.; et al. Effects of Steroids and Tocilizumab on the Immune Response Profile of Patients with COVID-19-Associated ARDS Requiring or Not Veno-Venous Extracorporeal Membrane Oxygenation. *Membranes* **2021**, *11*, 603. [CrossRef]
44. Liu, J.; Shu, Y.; Zhu, F.; Feng, B.; Zhang, Z.; Liu, L.; Wang, G. Comparative efficacy and safety of combination therapy with high-dose sulbactam or colistin with additional antibacterial agents for multiple drug-resistant and extensively drug-resistant *Acinetobacter baumannii* infections: A systematic review and network meta-analysis. *J. Glob. Antimicrob. Resist.* **2021**, *24*, 136–147. [PubMed]
45. Russo, A.; Bassetti, M.; Ceccarelli, G.; Carannante, N.; Losito, A.R.; Bartoletti, M.; Corcione, S.; Granata, G.; Santoro, A.; Giacobbe, D.R.; et al. ISGRI-SITA (Italian Study Group on Resistant Infections of the Società Italiana Terapia Antinfettiva) Bloodstream infections caused by carbapenem-resistant Acinetobacter baumannii: Clinical features, therapy and outcome from a multicenter study. *J. Infect.* **2019**, *79*, 130–138. [CrossRef] [PubMed]
46. Huttner, B.D.; Catho, G.; Pano-Pardo, J.R.; Pulcini, C.; Schouten, J. COVID-19: Don't neglect antimicrobial stewardship principles! *Clin. Microbiol. Infect.* **2020**, *26*, 808–810. [CrossRef] [PubMed]

Journal of
Clinical Medicine

MDPI

Article

Effectiveness of a Multifaced Antibiotic Stewardship Program: A Pre-Post Study in Seven Italian ICUs

Giulia Mandelli [1], Francesca Dore [1,2,*], Martin Langer [2,3], Elena Garbero [1,2], Laura Alagna [4], Andrea Bianchin [5], Rita Ciceri [2,6], Antonello Di Paolo [7], Tommaso Giani [8,9], Aimone Giugni [2,10], Andrea Gori [4,11,12], Ugo Lefons [13], Antonio Muscatello [4], Carlo Olivieri [2,14], Angelo Pan [15], Matteo Pedeferri [2,16], Marianna Rossi [17], Gian Maria Rossolini [8,9], Emanuele Russo [18], Daniela Silengo [2,19], Bruno Viaggi [2,20], Guido Bertolini [1] and Stefano Finazzi [1,2]

1 Istituto di Ricerche Farmacologiche Mario Negri IRCCS, 20156 Milano, Italy; giuliamandelli.bg@gmail.com (G.M.); elena.garbero@marionegri.it (E.G.); guido.bertolini@marionegri.it (G.B.); stefano.finazzi@marionegri.it (S.F.)
2 Associazione GiViTI—Gruppo Italiano per la Valutazione degli Interventi in Terapia Intensiva, 24020 Ranica, Italy; 10mlanger@gmail.com (M.L.); r.ciceri@asst-lecco.it (R.C.); aimonegiugni@gmail.com (A.G.); carlo.olivieri@aslvc.piemonte.it (C.O.); m.pedeferri@asst-lecco.it (M.P.); daniela.silengo@gmail.com (D.S.); bruno.viaggi@gmail.com (B.V.)
3 Emergency-Ong, 20128 Milano, Italy
4 Infectious Diseases Unit, Fondazione Istituto di Ricovero e Cura a Carattere Scientifico (IRCCS) Ca' Granda Ospedale Maggiore Policlinico, 20122 Milan, Italy; laura.alagna@gmail.com (L.A.); andrea.gori@unimi.it (A.G.); antonio.muscatello@policlinico.mi.it (A.M.)
5 Anesthesia and Intensive Care, Ospedale Civile San Valentino di Montebelluna, 31044 Montebelluna, Italy; andbia@libero.it
6 Anesthesia and Intensive Care, Ospedale Alessandro Manzoni di Lecco, 23900 Lecco, Italy
7 Department of Clinical and Experimental Medicine, Università di Pisa, 56126 Pisa, Italy; antonello.dipaolo@unipi.it
8 Department of Experimental and Clinical Medicine, Università di Firenze, 50134 Firenze, Italy; tommaso.giani@unifi.it (T.G.); gianmaria.rossolini@unifi.it (G.M.R.)
9 Clinical Microbiology and Virology Unit, Azienda Ospedaliero Universitaria Careggi, 50134 Firenze, Italy
10 Department of Intensive Care and Emergency Medical Services, Ospedale Maggiore, 40133 Bologna, Italy
11 Department of Pathophysiology and Transplantation, Università degli Studi di Milano, 20122 Milan, Italy
12 Centre for Multidisciplinary Research in Health Science (MACH), Università degli Studi di Milano, 20122 Milan, Italy
13 Anesthesia and Intensive Care, Ospedale Alta Val d'Elsa di Poggibonsi, 53036 Poggibonsi, Italy; ugo.lefons@uslsudest.toscana.it
14 Anesthesia and Intensive Care, Ospedale Sant'Andrea, ASL VC Vercelli, 13100 Vercelli, Italy
15 Infectious Diseases Unit, Istituti Ospitalieri di Cremona, 26100 Cremona, Italy; angelo.pan@asst-cremona.it
16 Anesthesia and Intensive Care, Presidio Ospedaliero San Leopoldo Mandić, 23807 Merate, Italy
17 Division of Infectious Diseases, "San Gerardo" Hospital, University of Milano-Bicocca, 20900 Monza, Italy; marianna.rossi@asst-monza.it
18 Anesthesia and Intensive Care, Ospedale Maurizio Bufalini di Cesena, 47521 Cesena, Italy; lelegaiola@gmail.com
19 Anesthesia and Intensive Care, Ospedale San Giovanni Bosco, 10154 Turin, Italy
20 Neuro Intensive Care Unit, Department of Anesthesiology, Azienda Ospedaliero Universitaria Careggi, 50134 Firenze, Italy
* Correspondence: francesca.dore@marionegri.it

Citation: Mandelli, G.; Dore, F.; Langer, M.; Garbero, E.; Alagna, L.; Bianchin, A.; Ciceri, R.; Di Paolo, A.; Giani, T.; Giugni, A.; et al. Effectiveness of a Multifaced Antibiotic Stewardship Program: A Pre-Post Study in Seven Italian ICUs. *J. Clin. Med.* **2022**, *11*, 4409. https://doi.org/10.3390/jcm11154409

Academic Editors: Luca Brazzi and Giorgia Montrucchio

Received: 19 May 2022
Accepted: 25 July 2022
Published: 28 July 2022

Abstract: Multidrug resistance has become a serious threat for health, particularly in hospital-acquired infections. To improve patients' safety and outcomes while maintaining the efficacy of antimicrobials, complex interventions are needed involving infection control and appropriate pharmacological treatments in antibiotic stewardship programs. We conducted a multicenter pre-post study to assess the impact of a stewardship program in seven Italian intensive care units (ICUs). Each ICU was visited by a multidisciplinary team involving clinicians, microbiologists, pharmacologists, infectious disease specialists, and data scientists. Interventions were targeted according to the characteristics of each unit. The effect of the program was measured with a panel of indicators computed with data from the MargheritaTre electronic health record. The median duration of empirical therapy decreased from 5.6 to 4.6 days and the use of quinolones dropped from 15.3% to 6%, both $p < 0.001$. The proportion of multi-drug-resistant bacteria (MDR) in ICU-acquired infections fell from 57.7% to 48.8%. ICU mortality and length of stay remained unchanged, indicating that reducing antibiotic administration did not harm patients' safety. This study shows that our stewardship program successfully improved the management of infections. This suggests that policy makers should tackle multidrug resistance with a multidisciplinary approach based on continuous monitoring and personalised interventions.

Keywords: antibiotic stewardship; multidrug resistance; intensive care units; healthcare-associated infections; infection control; electronic health record; education in medicine; appropriateness of antibiotic

1. Introduction

The efficacy of antimicrobials still saves the vast majority of patients suffering from bacterial or fungal infections. However, their use, overuse and mainly inappropriate use in and outside hospitals, as well as in livestock, favours the emergence of resistance. Resistant bacterial species threaten health and cause related morbidity and even mortality [1]. This has become a general emergency in hospitals and in general medical practice—although with significant geographical differences [2]. However, it is recognised that judicious use of antimicrobials is a cornerstone of the containment of multidrug resistance (MDR) [3].

Antibiotic stewardship programs (ASPs) are accepted worldwide as a must to improve patients' safety and outcomes, while maintaining the efficacy of antimicrobials by withholding the selective pressure driving antibiotic resistance (ABR) [4]. ASP comprises a bundle of interventions to improve several aspects of a complex decision-making process [5] involving organisation, prevention of transmission, diagnosis of infection, handling of microbiological investigations, optimisation of drug prescriptions [6], and duration of treatments.

There is general agreement on the urgent need for effective ASP, the best bundle composition, and the best way to implement these programs and to maintain the benefit over time. Most published stewardship programs, using very different methods, report success in achieving specific goals [7–14]. However, better management of infections calls for the design and achievement of several goals: reduction of the circulation and transmission of MDR [15] microorganisms and more appropriate use of drugs (sparing of carbapenems, limitation of quinolones and other broad-spectrum drugs, and appropriate site, dose, and duration of treatments).

Intensive care units (ICUs) present unique challenges for ASP due to their crucial position in the chain of antibiotic resistance: they admit critical and chronically ill patients frequently colonised by MDR microorganisms, transferred from hospital wards and nursing homes [16]. ICU doctors use antimicrobials generously, and return survivors with a greater or even unit-acquired MDR burden to the hospital and the community [17]. However, ICU personnel, having experienced how difficult it is to treat patients with MDR infections, do frequently pay closer attention to the MDR problem. ASPs have often been optimised in ICUs in recent years, with attempts also to develop the multidisciplinary aspect by including infectious diseases, microbiologists, and pharmacists in the projects.

In 2017 the Italian Group for the valuation of Intervention in Intensive Care Units (GIViTI, giviti@marionegri.it) started a multi-ICU project to control antibiotic resistance through a complex peer-to-peer intervention and extended monitoring with a common electronic health record (EHR), MargheritaTre (M3) [18] as a potential continuous antibiotic-stewardship tool.

The aim of this before/after project, intended as a pilot study, was to assess the efficacy of an ASP in a multicenter study. Specific goals of the ASP were reduction of the overall antibiotic pressure, sparing of the essential anti-MDR-drugs (e.g., carbapenems, colistin, linezolid), reduction of the use of quinolones, optimisation of drug administration, and improvement of appropriateness of antibiotic treatment. Appropriateness was assessed across several dimensions, focusing on infections with valid diagnostic specimens, microbiological diagnoses and pharmacologic properties as tissue penetration of the prescribed drugs. These actions, together with prevention of transmission, should yield the very ambitious achievement of reducing MDR infections. Considering the complexity of such a project, the ASP intervention was designed by a multidisciplinary team and agreed with the representatives of the participating ICUs.

The performance of each center was evaluated through a set of indicators designed to monitor several dimensions in the management of infections. The ASP interventions were tailored to each ICU on the basis of data collected during the first year of the project (before the intervention) and discussed with a panel of experts at on-site visits. The impact of the ASP over the year of observation was assessed by comparing the values of the indicators before and after the intervention. A further year of observation was planned to verify how long the benefits, if any, lasted.

2. Methods

2.1. Study Design

We ran a multicenter pre-post study to assess the impact of a stewardship program in ICUs. The program was based on a plenary meeting with representatives from ICUs and on-site audits. The impact of the program was measured by comparison of a panel of indicators computed before and after the intervention.

2.2. Participating Units

Participation in the study was voluntary, but limited to units working with the software M3, integrated with the laboratory information system. M3 is an EHR developed by a multidisciplinary team involving IT specialists, researchers, physicians, and nurses from the GiViTI network. It was designed to support clinical practice in ICUs and ensure high-quality data for research purposes [18]. M3 is property of Istituto di Ricerche Farmacologiche Mario Negri IRCCS (Milano, Italy) and GiViTI (Ranica, Italy).

2.3. Study Population

The study population comprised all patients admitted to seven general Italian ICUs of different sizes and case-mix. The study took place between January 2017 and February 2020 and had 12 months of data collection (see the Supplementary Materials for the list of ICUs and their characteristics).

2.4. Data Collection and Management

All data (clinical and microbiological diagnoses, laboratory tests, and treatments) were automatically acquired from the M3 EHR, without further intervention of the ICU physicians, limiting the risk of biases.

Information in M3 is primarily stored in structured or partially structured form to facilitate data analysis. Automatic services import patients' parameters and results of chemical and microbiological tests from monitors, ventilators, blood–gas analyser devices, and from the hospital information systems. M3 stores patients' data in a local PostgreSQL database in each hospital. Data are then encrypted and transferred in pseudonymised form to a server at the GiViTI coordinating center at the Mario Negri Institute for Pharmacological Research.

For this project we extracted the following variables from M3 databases: present-at-admission or ICU-acquired infection, site of infection, microbiological diagnosis and sensitivity pattern, where available, antimicrobials employed (drug, start and end dates of treatment, drug combinations), the rationale for antibiotic prescription (prophylaxis, targeted or empirical therapy), and length of ICU stay.

2.5. Phases of the Project

The study was coordinated and monitored by a study board nominated by the GiViTI steering committee. The members of the board were chosen for their expertise in critical care medicine, infectious diseases, clinical microbiology, and data science. The board defined the project's specific objectives and designed all the phases of the intervention.

Definition of the indicators: The study board designed all indicators to measure several dimensions related to the management of infections in ICUs (resistance patterns of the isolated microorganisms to drug classes, appropriateness of drug use, clinical decisions). When needed, the EHR M3 was modified to collect the variables employed to calculate those indicators.

Plenary session: A kick-off meeting was organised with representatives of the ICUs (nurses, intensivists, microbiologists, infectious disease specialists, pharmacists/pharmacologists) to share the objectives of the project, to describe its phases, and to recall and discuss standard strategies for infection control in the ICU and what is known to limit the emergence of antimicrobial resistance. This course was structured with plenary lectures and workgroups based on case records extracted from the EHR of the ICUs. The indicators to describe and quantify the measured data were discussed in this meeting.

To build a common multidisciplinary background, the topics discussed in the meeting aimed to update knowledge about risk stratification, diagnosis of infection, antibiotic prescription for community- and hospital-acquired infections, PK/PD optimisation, interpretation of antibiotic sensitivity tests for classical and novel diagnostic technologies, communication strategies with the laboratories, and information from biomarkers. The importance of environmental cleanliness and prevention of transmission were stressed as fundamental issues

On-site visits and follow up: All ICUs were visited between October 2018 and February 2019 by experienced members of the study board. The multidisciplinary visiting team involved an intensivist, a clinical microbiologist, an infectious disease specialist, and a data scientist from the coordinating team. Each visit lasted a whole day. The morning was dedicated to visiting the ICU and the microbiology laboratory to study the organisation of clinical activities and the decision-making. In the afternoon, pre-intervention data were evaluated, and critical aspects were identified and discussed. In a final de-briefing, the ICU members and the peers agreed on and fixed the goals to be achieved in one year. During this year each ICU could consult the clinical experts.

Final evaluation of the results: One year after the visit data from each center were processed and the indicators computed, each center received a report comparing its own performance to all the other ICUs.

The results were presented in a GiViTI meeting organised in online format due to COVID-19 restrictions in Italy.

2.6. Outcomes

The success of the stewardship program was evaluated through the following indicators. Mortality and ICU length of stay were used as safety parameters to make sure that the intervention did not harm patients.

2.6.1. Frequency of Patients with MDR Infections

Ratio of patients with at least one infection due to MDR bacteria according to the definition of Ref. [15] to the total number of infected patients. This endpoint was stratified by infections present at ICU admission or acquired during the ICU stay. Infections whose symptoms appeared during the first 48 h in the ICU were considered infections at admission.

2.6.2. Median Duration of Empirical Therapy and Prophylaxis

Kaplan–Meier curves were built to assess the duration of empirical therapies and prophylaxis (antimicrobial treatments aiming to avoid infections, including perioperative prophylaxis), censoring patients with ongoing therapies at discharge (see Supplementary Materials).

2.6.3. Inappropriateness of Antibiotics by Penetration into the Site of Infection

Ratio of inappropriate antibiotic therapies regarding tissue penetration to the number of antibiotics prescribed, based on a recent systematic review [19]. An antibiotic is considered inappropriate when it cannot reach the site of the infection.

2.6.4. Inappropriateness of Antibiotics by Microorganism Resistance Pattern

Ratio of inappropriate antibiotic therapies to the number of antibiotics prescribed. An antibiotic is considered as inappropriate if the bacteria causing the infection are intrinsically resistant [20] or resistant according to susceptibility tests [21–24].

2.6.5. Use of Fluoroquinolone Antibiotics

Proportion of patients who received at least one fluoroquinolone.

2.6.6. Inappropriate Prescriptions of Carbapenems

Ratio of inappropriate prescriptions of carbapenems to the total number of treatments with these drugs. Treatment with carbapenems is considered inappropriate when the microorganism causing the infection was responsive to other molecules with a more limited spectrum or anti-MDR specificity such as penicillin or cephalosporins.

2.6.7. Inappropriate Prescriptions of Colistin

Ratio of inappropriate prescriptions of colistin to the total number of treatments with these drugs. Treatment with colistin is considered inappropriate when the microorganism causing the infection was responsive to penicillin, cephalosporins, and carbapenems.

2.6.8. Inappropriate Prescriptions of Linezolid

Ratio of inappropriate prescriptions of linezolid to the total number of linezolid therapies. Empirical therapies in patients with acute renal failure were considered appropriate. Therapies in patients with SNC infection by Gram + bacteria or any infection due to MRSA or VRE were deemed appropriate.

The board of experts used three additional indicators to condense the results (before and after) in each ICU concerning patients' outcomes and drugs used.

- Antibiotic pressure: Proportion of days of ICU stay when patients received any antibiotic therapy.
- Average ICU length of stay.
- ICU mortality.

2.7. Statistical Analysis

Categorical variables are reported as frequency and percentage, continuous variables as mean and standard deviation (SD) or median and interquartile range (IQR), as appropriate.

Chi-squared and Wilcoxon rank-sum tests were applied to compare proportions and distributions of continuous variables, respectively, with a significance level of 0.05.

To take into account stratification by ICU, the results of the indicators before and after the intervention were compared using Cochran–Mantel–Haenszel, stratified Mann–Whitney, and stratified log-rank tests for proportions, distribution of continuous variables, and Kaplan–Meier curves, as appropriate, with a significance level of 0.05.

All analyses were done with R, version 3.6 (R Core Team, R Foundation for Statistical Computing, Vienna, Austria).

3. Results

The indicators were evaluated for data collected in 2018 on 2901 patients to assess the performance of the seven ICUs before the ASP intervention. The program's efficacy was assessed by comparing the same indicators on data collected for a whole year after the site visits for 3389 patients. The patients' main characteristics are reported in Table 1.

The indicators computed in the pre- and post-intervention phases are compared in Table 2. Improvement was obtained on the frequency of infections caused by MDR bacteria (39.5% post-intervention vs 44.9% pre-intervention), especially for ICU-acquired infections (48.8% vs. 57.7%). The frequency of MDR in infections on admission and acquired in ICU for each center are plotted in Figure 1a,b, before (dashed) and after (solid) the ASP intervention. The horizontal lines indicate the overall average. Although the Cochran–Mantel–Haenszel tests are not significant, the changes are substantial and the percentage of MDR in ICU-acquired infection decreased in all but one of the participating ICUs.

Table 1. Descriptive table (pre-/post-) main demographics, comorbidities, infections present at ICU admission and infections acquired during ICU stay. Significant levels are indicated as * $p < 0.05$, ** $p < 0.01$, *** $p < 0.001$.

	Total (6290)	Pre-Intervention (2901)	Post-Intervention (3389)	*p*-Value	
Median Age (Q1, Q3)	66 (51, 77)	67 (52, 77)	65 (51, 76)	0.003	***
Male	3816 (60.7%)	1755 (60.5%)	2061 (60.8%)	0.80	
ICU Outcome	1011 (16.1%)	471 (16.2%)	540 (15.9%)	0.75	
		Comorbidities			
Hypertension	2818 (48.9%)	1321 (48.4%)	1497 (49.4%)	0.48	
Severe Obesity (BMI > 35)	979 (17.0%)	440 (16.1%)	539 (17.8%)	0.10	
Arrythmia	839 (14.6%)	391 (14.3%)	448 (14.8%)	0.64	
Type 2 Diabetes	1018 (17.7%)	460 (16.9%)	558 (18.4%)	0.13	
BPCO	840 (14.6%)	401 (14.7%)	439 (14.5%)	0.81	
Tumor	683 (11.9%)	348 (12.8%)	335 (11.0%)	0.05	*
Myocardial Infarction	531 (9.2%)	241 (8.8%)	290 (9.6%)	0.34	
Moderate/Severe Renal Failure	450 (7.8%)	193 (7.1%)	257 (8.5%)	0.05	*
NYHA 2, 3	450 (7.8%)	208 (7.6%)	242 (8.0%)	0.62	
Vasculopathy	409 (7.1%)	239 (8.8%)	170 (5.6%)	<0.001	***
No comorbidities	1069 (18.6%)	552 (20.2%)	517 (17.1%)	0.002	**
		Infections on admission			
Pneumonia	579 (9.7%)	286 (10.6%)	293 (9.0%)	0.04	*
Clinical sepsis	226 (3.8%)	98 (3.6%)	128 (3.9%)	0.56	
Peritonitis	241 (4.1%)	118 (4.4%)	123 (3.8%)	0.24	
Urinary tract infections	116 (1.9%)	50 (1.9%)	66 (2.0%)	0.64	
Skin/soft-tissue Infection	102 (1.7%)	45 (1.7%)	57 (1.8%)	0.81	

Table 1. *Cont.*

	Total (6290)	Pre-Intervention (2901)	Post-Intervention (3389)	p-Value
No infections	4488 (75.4%)	2009 (74.6%)	2479 (76.1%)	0.16
		ICU acquired infections		
Pneumonia	599 (9.5%)	285 (9.8%)	314 (9.3%)	0.45
Lower respiratory tract infection	211 (3.4%)	103 (3.6%)	108 (3.2%)	0.43
Clinical Sepsis	100 (1.6%)	49 (1.7%)	51 (1.5%)	0.560
Primary bloodstream infection	128 (2.0%)	60 (2.1%)	68 (2.0%)	0.86
Urinary tract infection	95 (1.5%)	39 (1.3%)	56 (1.7%)	0.32

Table 2. Endpoints with % pre-/post- (aggregated) and p-values for all indicators. Significant levels are indicated as * $p < 0.05$, *** $p < 0.001$.

	Pre-Intervention	Post-Intervention	p-Value	
Frequency of patients with MDR infections (N/D)	44.9% (315/701)	39.5% (305/772)	0.11	
On admission (N/D)	27.7% (131/473)	25.5% (135/529	0.59	
ICU acquired (N/D)	57.7% (203/352)	48.8% (189/387)	0.09	
Median (IQR) duration of empirical therapy (D)	5.6 days (1275)	4.6 days (1406)	<0.001	***
Median duration of prophylaxis (D)	2.3 days (589)	2.0 days (584)	0.06	
Inappropriateness of antibiotics by penetration into the site of infection (N/D)	2.3% (49/2117)	1.9% (49/2619)	0.26	
Inappropriateness of antibiotics by microorganism resistance pattern in empirical therapy (N/D)	16.2% (57/351)	17.3% (67/387)	0.84	
Inappropriateness of antibiotics by microorganism resistance pattern in targeted therapy (N/D)	3.8% (19/507)	4.8% (29/606)	0.29	
Use of quinolones (N/D)	15.3% (251/1637)	6.0% (105/1737)	<0.001	***
Inappropriate prescriptions of carbapenems in empirical therapy (N/D)	45.2% (19/42)	36.9% (24/65)	0.51	
Inappropriate prescriptions of carbapenems in targeted therapy (N/D)	36.7% (18/49)	55.3% (42/76)	0.07	
Inappropriate prescriptions of colistin in targeted therapy	27.6% (8/29)	40% (2/5)	0.61	
Inappropriate prescriptions of linezolid (N/D)	54.9% (82/150)	69.8% (127/182)	0.01	*
Average ICU Length of stay (D)	5.5 days (2901)	5.4 days (3389)	0.07	
ICU Mortality (N/D)	16.2% (471/2901)	15.9% (540/3389)	0.54	

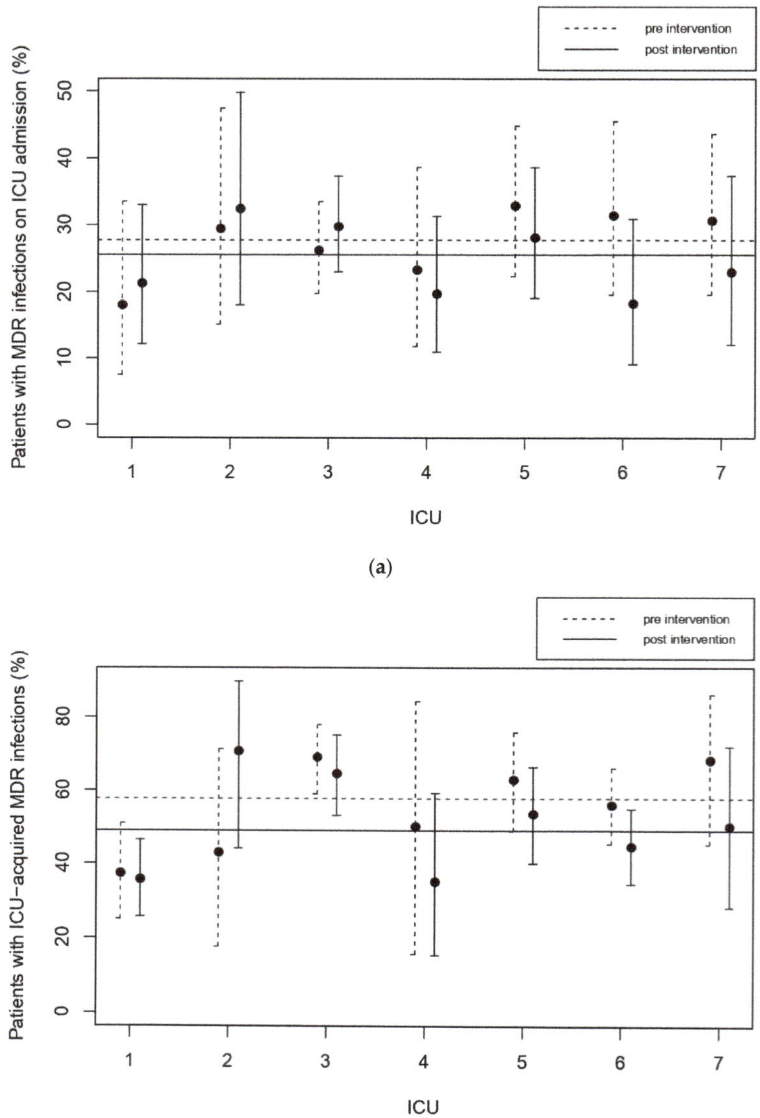

(**a**)

(**b**)

Figure 1. %MDR on admission (panel (**a**)) and %MDR in ICU-acquired infections (>48 h, panel (**b**)) for the participating centers, pre- (dashed line) and post-intervention (solid line). The horizontal line indicates the average.

The median duration of empirical therapy and prophylaxis was reduced from 5.6 to 4.6 days ($p < 0.001$) and from 2.3 to 2.0 days ($p = 0.06$), respectively. The median duration of empirical therapy before the intervention ranged from about 4 to 8 days in the seven ICUs. This decreased in all the ICUs, significantly in four of them (Figure 2a). Regarding prophylaxis, the behaviour of the ICUs differed widely (Figure 2b). The two ICUs with the longest durations before the intervention improved their performance, coming close to the average of all the centers. The duration of prophylaxis significantly increased only in one ICU, nonetheless remaining well below the average.

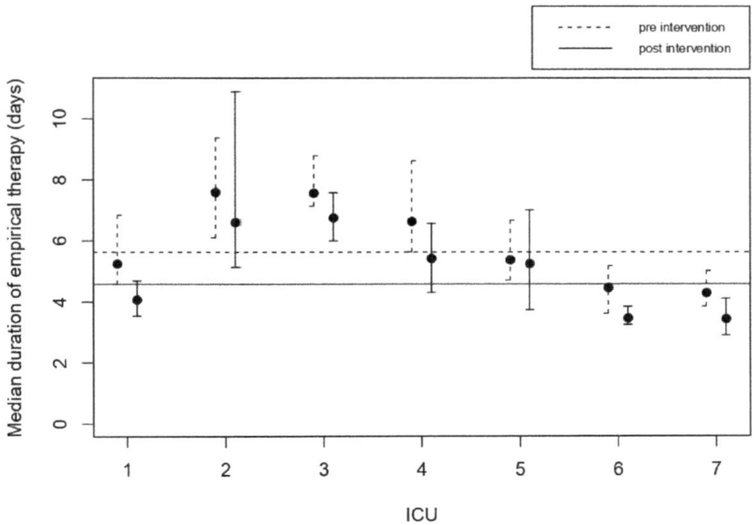

(**a**)

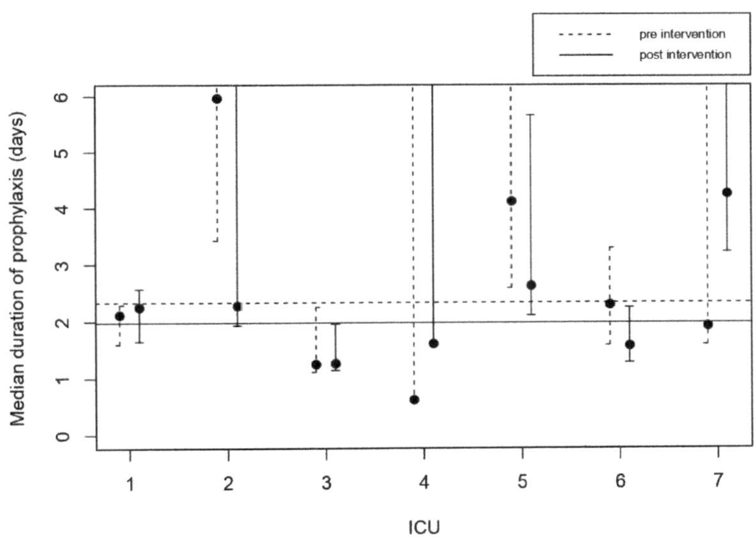

(**b**)

Figure 2. Median duration of empirical therapy (**a**) and prophylaxis (**b**) for the participating centers, pre- (dashed line) and post-intervention (solid line). The horizontal line indicates the average. The use of quinolones more than halved. Before the intervention 15.3% of patients needing antibiotics received quinolones. This decreased to 6.0% after the intervention ($p < 0.001$). Quinolones were used for about 10% to 30% of patients in the seven ICUs. Its usage in all the units decreased in both value and variability, ranging from about 3% to 10% (Figure 3a).

The only indicator that significantly increased was the use of linezolid, though with a limited number of prescriptions. After our ASP, 69.8% of linezolid prescriptions were inappropriate (as defined in Section 2), while 54.9% were considered inappropriate before the intervention. This worsened in more than half of the centers (Figure 3b), but the confidence intervals are quite wide since only a few patients received linezolid.

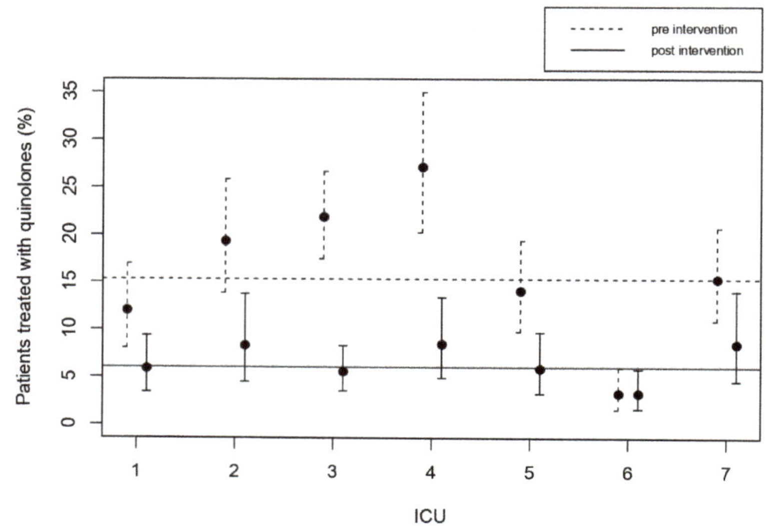

(a)

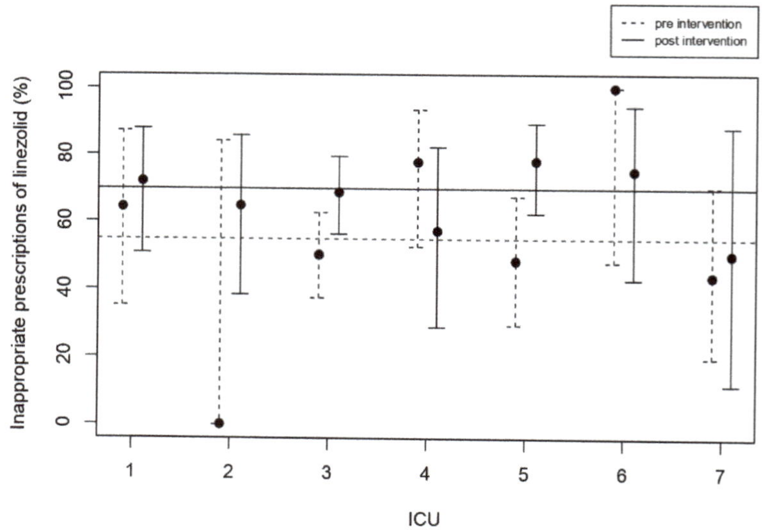

(b)

Figure 3. Use of quinolones (**a**) and inappropriate prescriptions of linezolid (**b**) for the participating centers, pre- (dashed line) and post-intervention (solid line). The horizontal line indicates the average.

How far appropriateness is concerned, 16,2% and 17,3% of empirical, and 3,8% and 4.8% of targeted treatments were considered inappropriate according to our definitions and no pre/post change could be found (Table 2).

The average length of stay increased (not significantly) from 5.4 to 5.5 days ($p = 0.07$) and mortality remained unchanged (from 16.2% to 15.9%).

The other indicators did not change significantly. They are plotted in the Supplementary Materials.

4. Discussion

Continuous education and monitoring and improvement of the quality of care in ICUs are the primary missions of the GiViTI group. Given the lasting interest in the epidemiology and reduction of infectious complications in critically ill patients [25], an ASP study was mandatory. The objectives of an ASP are the containment of infections, better use of antimicrobials, and reduction of the emergence and spread of MDR bacteria. Although these goals are universally recognised, standardised methods for their implementation and monitoring are far from being defined yet.

Here, we report a pilot ASP that was education- and culture-based, with no additional workload or formal protocols for healthcare workers. Its implementation was adapted to the different operating conditions of each ICU. The indicators used to monitor the ICU performance are simple, easy to understand and offer a possible tool for continuous surveillance.

Monitoring was made easier by taking data directly from the EHR M3, thus minimising the risk of bias due to the manual input into an ad hoc case report form. Standardised indicators addressing several items in the ASP were automatically computed from M3 data: admission of infected and MDR-infected patients, ICU-related acquisition of MDR infection, duration of antimicrobial treatments (targeted, empirical, or prophylactic), and number of treatments with specific antimicrobials (carbapenems, colistin, quinolones, and linezolid).

Outcomes such as the length of stay and mortality cannot be seen as indicators of efficacy but as an attempt to monitor safety. The possibility of benchmarking results in time with a before/after analysis and among units stimulates them to improve their performance and shows that improvements are possible in clinical practice.

Seven units participated in our study on a voluntary basis. The kick-off meeting of the project gave the opportunity to update clinical knowledge and governance policies. The site visits established personal relationships with the experts and from the discussion of data the specific weak points of each unit could be identified to set individual goals.

Data collected before the intervention from 2901 patients (Table 1) showed large baseline differences among centers. This testifies to the wide diversity in patients' case mix and clinical behaviour as reported in Ref. [2].

The results of the project were positive for the majority of indicators, apparently without causing patients any harm. As in other ASPs [5,8–11,13,26,27], there were reductions in antibiotic prescriptions (especially quinolones), treatment duration, and MDR emergence.

As quinolones are considered as facilitators of MDR [28–32], the drastic reduction of their prescriptions confirms the willingness to improve therapeutic strategies based on scientific knowledge and compliance to protocols. Shorter durations of empirical treatments suggest more efficient management of microbiological samples, from withdrawal to reporting of sensitivity tests. The marked reduction of ICU-acquired MDR infections, although globally non-significant and with quite large differences between centers, illustrates a general improvement in the management of infected patients, regarding either antibiotic prescriptions or infection control.

No before/after changes could be found in the appropriateness issues (Table 2). Our expectations were probably too ambitious and the methodology and definitions not able to detect differences in the prescribing behaviour.

Non-significant changes were observed in the use of carbapenems, and a specific study may be necessary to understand this result more in fully.

The original plan of the study included one more year of observation in 2020 to test the "survival" of improved clinical practice, but unfortunately the COVID pandemic changed the case mix and the ICU work so deeply that comparisons would be meaningless.

Nonetheless, what have we learned from this experience? The enthusiastic acceptance and collaboration of clinicians delegated by each ICU as project contact persons underline the intensivists' interest in improving clinical practice.

In view of the voluntary nature of the project, it was hard to engage colleagues not directly involved in the ASP. In a few ICUs, local site visits were limited because of work shifts, holidays, or lack of interest. The results of the project are more effective and enduring when the ASP message and the need for its implementation are shared among the whole ICU staff.

The ICU is a key node in the complex hospital network of players involved in the management of infections. However, an ASP would not be effective if devoted only to ICU physicians and nurses. For this reason, we also invited on-site microbiologists, pharmacists, and infectious disease specialists to participate at the site visits and encouraged the creation of multidisciplinary teams.

Our pilot project was very resource-consuming: we could never offer it to the approximately 200 units associated with GiViTI. To extend the program to other ICUs, we would have to identify which parts of our project were essential and which could be resized, saving workforce and time.

Furthermore, the medical community has to take account of the terrible impact of the SARS-CoV-2 pandemic on the use of antibiotics in the population, inside and outside hospitals and ICUs [33]. ASPs will be urgently and widely necessary, at least to return to the basic concepts of proper antibiotic prescription of the "pre-COVID" era. Similarly, the reduction in MDR infections needs to be rapidly transferred into real COVID-19 life, since in Italy there has been a significant increase of these pathogens. Hopefully our experience will be helpful.

Limitations of the Study

The main limitation of the study is the lack of the second year of monitoring the ASP indicators to see if the positive effects were just a "study-related" benefit or it really changed the use of antimicrobial drugs. Most of our participating units are in northern Italy, and most of them became COVID ICUs with a completely different case mix and organisation.

Moreover, the number of participating ICUs was limited. Unfortunately, at that time, few ICUs met the necessary conditions for participation: interest in the study, use of M3 as the EHR, and integration of M3 with the laboratory. For these reasons, we downgraded our study to a pilot study, which, however, gave a considerable amount of important information.

5. Conclusions

Our ASP adopted a multidisciplinary approach involving clinicians, microbiologists, pharmacologists, infectious disease specialists, and data scientists. It successfully reduced antibiotic consumption and MDR, without risking patient safety. Simple indicators, which can easily be updated to the newer drugs and different patient populations, were automatically computed from common EHR, helping to monitor ASP data.

The feasibility and the success of this multicenter ASP should now encourage healthcare policy makers to consider that "where there's a will, there's a way".

Supplementary Materials: The following supporting information can be downloaded at: https://www.mdpi.com/article/10.3390/jcm11154409/s1. 1. List of ICUs; 2. ICU characteristics; 3. Survival analysis for median duration of antibiotics treatments; 4. Indicators—comparison among ICUs. (a) Frequency of patients with MDR infections. (b) Inappropriateness of antibiotics by penetration into the site of infection. (c) Inappropriateness of antibiotics by microorganism resistance pattern in empirical therapy. (d) Inappropriateness of antibiotics by microorganism resistance pattern in targeted therapy. (e) Use of carbapenems. (f) Average ICU Length of stay. (g) ICU Mortality.

Author Contributions: Conceptualization, G.M., S.F., G.B. and B.V.; methodology, S.F. and G.M.; statistical analysis, S.F. and G.M.; investigation, definition of indicators and on-site visits, S.F., G.M., G.B., M.L., B.V., A.D.P., A.G. (Andrea Gori), C.O., A.P., G.M.R., D.S., T.G., L.A., M.R. and A.M.; implementation of stewardship intervention, D.S., R.C., A.G. (Aimone Giugni), U.L., E.R., A.B. and M.P.; data curation, G.M.; writing—draft preparation, S.F., G.M., M.L. and F.D.; review & editing, S.F., G.M., F.D., G.B., M.L., B.V., A.D.P., A.G. (Andrea Gori), C.O., A.P., G.M.R., D.S., T.G., L.A., M.R. and A.M.; project administration, G.M. and E.G. All authors have read and agreed to the published version of the manuscript.

Funding: This research was funded by MSD, ALIFAXe Thermo Fisher Scientific through an unconditional contribution.

Institutional Review Board Statement: The project was conducted as an educational program to improve the quality of care. Data collection with the electronic health record, *MargheritaTre* received the approval from the Ethics Committee of the Coordinating Center, Ospedale Maggiore di Bologna (ethic code 17164).

Data Availability Statement: Data can be accessed upon request and under appropriate data sharing agreement.

Conflicts of Interest: The authors declare no conflict of interest influencing the representation or interpretation of reported research results.

References

1. French, G.L. Clinical Impact and Relevance of Antibiotic Resistance. *Adv. Drug Deliv. Rev.* **2005**, *57*, 1514–1527. [CrossRef] [PubMed]
2. World Health Organization. *WHO Report on Surveillance of Antibiotic Consumption: 2016–2018 Early Implementation*; World Health Organization: Geneva, Switzerland, 2018.
3. Livermore, D.M. Minimising Antibiotic Resistance. *Lancet Infect. Dis.* **2005**, *5*, 450–459. [CrossRef]
4. Davey, P.; Brown, E.; Charani, E.; Fenelon, L.; Gould, I.M.; Holmes, A.; Ramsay, C.R.; Wiffen, P.J.; Wilcox, M. Interventions to Improve Antibiotic Prescribing Practices for Hospital Inpatients. *Cochrane Database Syst. Rev.* **2013**, *4*, CD003543.
5. Tamma, P.D.; Miller, M.A.; Cosgrove, S.E. Rethinking How Antibiotics Are Prescribed: Incorporating the 4 Moments of Antibiotic Decision Making into Clinical Practice. *JAMA* **2019**, *321*, 139–140. [CrossRef] [PubMed]
6. Klein, E.Y.; Milkowska-Shibata, M.; Tseng, K.K.; Sharland, M.; Gandra, S.; Pulcini, C.; Laxminarayan, R. Assessment of WHO Antibiotic Consumption and Access Targets in 76 Countries, 2000–15: An Analysis of Pharmaceutical Sales Data. *Lancet Infect. Dis.* **2021**, *21*, 107–115. [CrossRef]
7. Zhang, Y.-Z.; Singh, S. Antibiotic Stewardship Programmes in Intensive Care Units: Why, How, and Where Are They Leading Us. *World J. Crit. Care Med.* **2015**, *4*, 13. [CrossRef] [PubMed]
8. Taggart, L.R.; Leung, E.; Muller, M.P.; Matukas, L.M.; Daneman, N. Differential Outcome of an Antimicrobial Stewardship Audit and Feedback Program in Two Intensive Care Units: A Controlled Interrupted Time Series Study. *BMC Infect. Dis.* **2015**, *15*, 480. [CrossRef] [PubMed]
9. Álvarez-Lerma, F.; Grau, S.; Echeverría-Esnal, D.; Martínez-Alonso, M.; Gracia-Arnillas, M.P.; Horcajada, J.P.; Masclans, J.R. A Before-and-after Study of the Effectiveness of an Antimicrobial Stewardship Program in Critical Care. *Antimicrob. Agents Chemother.* **2018**, *62*, e01825-17. [CrossRef] [PubMed]
10. Thursky, K.A.; Buising, K.L.; Bak, N.; Macgregor, L.; Street, A.C.; Macintyre, C.R.; Presneill, J.J.; Cade, J.F.; Brown, G.V. Reduction of Broad-Spectrum Antibiotic Use with Computerized Decision Support in an Intensive Care Unit. *Int. J. Qual. Health Care* **2006**, *18*, 224–231. [CrossRef] [PubMed]
11. Leung, V.; Gill, S.; Sauve, J.; Walker, K.; Stumpo, C.; Powis, J. Growing a "Positive Culture" of Antimicrobial Stewardship in a Community Hospital. *Can. J. Hosp. Pharm.* **2011**, *64*, 314. [CrossRef] [PubMed]
12. Langford, B.J.; Beriault, D.; Schwartz, K.L.; Seah, J.; Pasic, M.D.; Cirone, R.; Chan, A.; Downing, M. A Real-World Assessment of Procalcitonin Combined with Antimicrobial Stewardship in a Community ICU. *J. Crit. Care* **2020**, *57*, 130–133. [CrossRef] [PubMed]
13. Wang, H.-Y.; Chiu, C.-H.; Huang, C.-T.; Cheng, C.-W.; Lin, Y.-J.; Hsu, Y.-J.; Chen, C.-H.; Deng, S.-T.; Leu, H.-S. Blood Culture-Guided de-Escalation of Empirical Antimicrobial Regimen for Critical Patients in an Online Antimicrobial Stewardship Programme. *Int. J. Antimicrob. Agents* **2014**, *44*, 520–527. [CrossRef] [PubMed]
14. Ramsamy, Y.; Muckart, D.J.J.; Han, K.S.S. Microbiological Surveillance and Antimicrobial Stewardship Minimise the Need for Ultrabroad-Spectrum Combination Therapy for Treatment of Nosocomial Infections in a Trauma Intensive Care Unit: An Audit of an Evidence-Based Empiric Antimicrobial Policy. *S. Afr. Med. J.* **2013**, *103*, 371–376. [CrossRef] [PubMed]

15. Magiorakos, A.-P.; Srinivasan, A.; Carey, R.B.; Carmeli, Y.; Falagas, M.E.; Giske, C.G.; Harbarth, S.; Hindler, J.F.; Kahlmeter, G.; Olsson-Liljequist, B. Multidrug-Resistant, Extensively Drug-Resistant and Pandrug-Resistant Bacteria: An International Expert Proposal for Interim Standard Definitions for Acquired Resistance. *Clin. Microbiol. Infect.* **2012**, *18*, 268–281. [CrossRef]
16. Doernberg, S.B.; Chambers, H.F. Antimicrobial Stewardship Approaches in the Intensive Care Unit. *Infect. Dis. Clin.* **2017**, *31*, 513–534. [CrossRef] [PubMed]
17. De Waele, J.J.; Akova, M.; Antonelli, M.; Canton, R.; Carlet, J.; De Backer, D.; Dimopoulos, G.; Garnacho-Montero, J.; Kesecioglu, J.; Lipman, J. Antimicrobial Resistance and Antibiotic Stewardship Programs in the ICU: Insistence and Persistence in the Fight against Resistance. A Position Statement from ESICM/ESCMID/WAAAR Round Table on Multi-Drug Resistance. *Intensive Care Med.* **2018**, *44*, 189–196. [CrossRef]
18. Finazzi, S.; Mandelli, G.; Garbero, E.; Mondini, M.; Trussardi, G.; Giardino, M.; Tavola, M.; Bertolini, G. Data Collection and Research with MargheritaTre. *Physiol. Meas.* **2018**, *39*, 084004. [CrossRef] [PubMed]
19. Finazzi, S.; Luci, G.; Olivieri, C.; Langer, M.; Mandelli, G.; Gori, A.; Viaggi, B.; Di Paolo, A. Tissue penetration of antimicrobials in intensive care unit patients: A systematic review—Part II. *Antibiotics* **2022**, *11*. *submitted*.
20. Leclercq, R.; Cantón, R.; Brown, D.F.; Giske, C.G.; Heisig, P.; MacGowan, A.P.; Mouton, J.W.; Nordmann, P.; Rodloff, A.C.; Rossolini, G.M. EUCAST Expert Rules in Antimicrobial Susceptibility Testing. *Clin. Microbiol. Infect.* **2013**, *19*, 141–160. [CrossRef]
21. The European Committee on Antimicrobial Susceptibility Testing. Breakpoint Tables for Interpretation of MICs and Zone Diameters, Version 8.1. 2018. Available online: http://www.eucast.org/Clinical_breakpoints/ (accessed on 20 May 2020).
22. The European Committee on Antimicrobial Susceptibility Testing. Breakpoint Tables for Interpretation of MICs and Zone Diameters, Version 9.0. 2019. Available online: http://www.eucast.or/Clinical_breakpoints/ (accessed on 20 May 2020).
23. CLSI. *Performance Standards for Antimicrobial Susceptibility Testing*, 28th ed.; CLSI Supplement M100; Wayne, P.A., Ed.; Clinical and Laboratory Standards Institute: Wayne, PA, USA, 2018.
24. CLSI. *Performance Standards for Antimicrobial Susceptibility Testing*, 29th ed.; CLSI Supplement M100; Wayne, P.A., Ed.; Clinical and Laboratory Standards Institute: Wayne, PA, USA, 2019.
25. Carlet, J.; Ali, A.B.; Chalfine, A. Epidemiology and Control of Antibiotic Resistance in the Intensive Care Unit. *Curr. Opin. Infect. Dis.* **2004**, *17*, 309–316. [CrossRef]
26. Apisarnthanarak, A.; Pinitchai, U.; Warachan, B.; Warren, D.K.; Khawcharoenporn, T.; Hayden, M.K. Effectiveness of Infection Prevention Measures Featuring Advanced Source Control and Environmental Cleaning to Limit Transmission of Extremely-Drug Resistant Acinetobacter Baumannii in a Thai Intensive Care Unit: An Analysis before and after Extensive Flooding. *Am. J. Infect. Control* **2014**, *42*, 116–121. [PubMed]
27. Frattari, A.; Savini, V.; Polilli, E.; Di Marco, G.; Lucisano, G.; Corridoni, S.; Spina, T.; Costantini, A.; Nicolucci, A.; Fazii, P. Control of Gram-Negative Multi-Drug Resistant Microorganisms in an Italian ICU: Rapid Decline as a Result of a Multifaceted Intervention, Including Conservative Use of Antibiotics. *Int. J. Infect. Dis.* **2019**, *84*, 153–162. [CrossRef] [PubMed]
28. Johnson, S.W.; Anderson, D.J.; May, D.B.; Drew, R.H. Utility of a Clinical Risk Factor Scoring Model in Predicting Infection with Extended-Spectrum β-Lactamase-Producing Enterobacteriaceae on Hospital Admission. *Infect. Control Hosp. Epidemiol.* **2013**, *34*, 385–392. [CrossRef] [PubMed]
29. Tumbarello, M.; Trecarichi, E.M.; Bassetti, M.; De Rosa, F.G.; Spanu, T.; Di Meco, E.; Losito, A.R.; Parisini, A.; Pagani, N.; Cauda, R. Identifying Patients Harboring Extended-Spectrum-β-Lactamase-Producing Enterobacteriaceae on Hospital Admission: Derivation and Validation of a Scoring System. *Antimicrob. Agents Chemother.* **2011**, *55*, 3485–3490. [CrossRef]
30. Tumbarello, M.; Trecarichi, E.M.; Tumietto, F.; Del Bono, V.; De Rosa, F.G.; Bassetti, M.; Losito, A.R.; Tedeschi, S.; Saffioti, C.; Corcione, S. Predictive Models for Identification of Hospitalized Patients Harboring KPC-Producing *Klebsiella pneumoniae*. *Antimicrob. Agents Chemother.* **2014**, *58*, 3514–3520. [CrossRef] [PubMed]
31. Van der Bij, A.K.; Pitout, J.D. The Role of International Travel in the Worldwide Spread of Multiresistant Enterobacteriaceae. *J. Antimicrob. Chemother.* **2012**, *67*, 2090–2100. [CrossRef] [PubMed]
32. Bassetti, M.; Carnelutti, A.; Peghin, M. Patient Specific Risk Stratification for Antimicrobial Resistance and Possible Treatment Strategies in Gram-Negative Bacterial Infections. *Expert Rev. Anti-Infect. Ther.* **2017**, *15*, 55–65. [CrossRef] [PubMed]
33. Mojica, M.F.; Rossi, M.-A.; Vila, A.J.; Bonomo, R.A. The Urgent Need for Metallo-β-Lactamase Inhibitors: An Unattended Global Threat. *Lancet Infect. Dis.* **2021**, *22*, e28–e34. [CrossRef]

Journal of
Clinical Medicine

MDPI

Article

Effectiveness of an Active and Continuous Surveillance Program for Intensive Care Units Infections Based on the EPIC III (Extended Prevalence of Infection in Intensive Care) Approach

Giorgia Montrucchio [1,2,*], Gabriele Sales [1,2], Giulia Catozzi [3], Stefano Bosso [4], Martina Scanu [2], Titty Vita Vignola [5], Andrea Costamagna [1,2], Silvia Corcione [6,7], Rosario Urbino [2], Claudia Filippini [1], Francesco Giuseppe De Rosa [6] and Luca Brazzi [1,2]

1 Department of Surgical Sciences, University of Turin, 10126 Turin, Italy; gabriele.sales@unito.it (G.S.); andrea.costamagna@unito.it (A.C.); claudia.filippini@unito.it (C.F.); luca.brazzi@unito.it (L.B.)
2 Department of Anaesthesia, Critical Care and Emergency, Città Della Salute e Della Scienza Hospital, Corso Dogliotti 14, 10126 Turin, Italy; martiscanu89@gmail.com (M.S.); rurbinocsst@gmail.com (R.U.)
3 Department of Health Sciences, University of Milan, 20122 Milan, Italy; giuliacatozzi.ds@gmail.com
4 Department of Anesthesiology and Critical Care, "Cardinal Massaia" Hospital, 14100 Asti, Italy; steo_bos@libero.it
5 Anesthesia and Intensive Care Unit, San Giovanni Bosco Hospital, 10154 Turin, Italy; tittyvitavignola@outlook.it
6 Department of Medical Sciences, Infectious Diseases, University of Turin, 10126 Turin, Italy; silvia.corcione@unito.it (S.C.); francescogiuseppe.derosa@unito.it (F.G.D.R.)
7 School of Medicine, Tufts University, Boston, MA 02111, USA
* Correspondence: giorgiagiuseppina.montrucchio@unito.it

Citation: Montrucchio, G.; Sales, G.; Catozzi, G.; Bosso, S.; Scanu, M.; Vignola, T.V.; Costamagna, A.; Corcione, S.; Urbino, R.; Filippini, C.; et al. Effectiveness of an Active and Continuous Surveillance Program for Intensive Care Units Infections Based on the EPIC III (Extended Prevalence of Infection in Intensive Care) Approach. *J. Clin. Med.* **2022**, *11*, 2482. https://doi.org/10.3390/jcm11092482

Academic Editor: Olivier Mimoz

Received: 17 March 2022
Accepted: 27 April 2022
Published: 28 April 2022

Abstract: We evaluated the effectiveness of the Extended Prevalence of Infection in Intensive Care (EPIC) III data collection protocol as an active surveillance tool in the eight Intensive Care Units (ICUs) of the Intensive and Critical Care Department of the University Hospital of Turin. A total of 435 patients were included in a six-day study over 72 ICU beds. 42% had at least one infection: 69% at one site, 26% at two sites and 5% at three or more sites. ICU-acquired infections were the most common (64%), followed by hospital-associated infections (22%) and community-acquired (20%), considering that each patient may have developed more than one infection type. 72% of patients were receiving at least one antibiotic: 48% for prophylaxis and 52% for treatment. Mortality, the length of ICU and hospital stays were 13%, 14 and 29 days, respectively, being all estimated to be significantly different in patients without and with infection (8% vs. 20%; 4 vs. 20 and 11 vs. 50 ($p < 0.001$). Our data confirm a high prevalence of infections, sepsis and the use of antimicrobials. The repeated punctual prevalence survey seems an effective method to carry out the surveillance of infections and the use of antimicrobials in the ICU. The use of the European Centre for Disease Prevention and Control (ECDC) definitions and the EPIC III protocol seems strategic to allow comparisons with national and international contexts.

Keywords: infections; intensive care unit; antimicrobial stewardship; infection control; drug resistance; bacterial; point prevalence study

1. Introduction

Infections are a major cause of admissions and prolonged stays in intensive care units (ICUs). They affect approximately 30% of patients, with large variations between different geographical regions [1–7], and they are the leading cause of death in non-cardiac ICUs, with still very high mortality rates and associated costs [8,9].

Sepsis and septic shock can complicate both community-acquired infections, which account for up to 70% of all cases of sepsis [8], and healthcare-associated infections (HAI), which would be mostly preventable by adequate infection prevention and control (IPC) measures [10–12].

Although extremely variable in the literature, data regarding the real prevalence of HAIs remains high in Europe (6.5%) [13,14], with values probably much higher in ICUs. Unfortunately, many articles do not report the differentiation between community and hospital-acquired sepsis, leading to a possible underestimation of the impact of HAIs, however potentially prevented in about 55% of cases by the implementation of multifaceted IPC interventions [15–17].

Epidemiological information on the underlying source of infections, associated microorganisms, treatment and outcomes are essential to identify gaps and optimize patient management. Unfortunately, although surveillance systems have been proposed at local [18] and international levels [19,20], adherence to them is not uniform in terms of both data collection and definitions [21], and this limits the comparability of the data over time. In particular, the integration between infection and/or colonization systematic data collection, control measures, and their application and evolution over time is complex. Moreover, data complexity does not allow their timely use, given the long processing and interpretation times, partially limiting the possibility of continuous and proactive surveillance. Another point to be considered is the lack of local comparisons, on a national or regional basis, capable of reflecting the specific characteristics of the population, the intensity of care, as well as the microbiological trend of the local ecology.

In this scenario, the use of punctual prevalence studies, which are more easily achievable and repeatable over time, has been proposed, especially in ICUs. Their validity and reliability, however, might be limited, given the method and timing of the data collection used [22].

Recently, a worldwide study [9] collected comprehensive data on the global epidemiology of ICU infections in 1150 centers in 88 countries, reporting that 54% of admitted patients had suspected or proven infection, 70% received at least one antibiotic, and Gram-negative bacteria were the predominant microorganisms (67%). One of the strengths of this study was the use of an exhaustive but essential data collection protocol, widely applicable in different contexts, which guaranteed great participation and reliability of the collected data.

As valid epidemiological data are needed to increase the awareness of the impact of infection among ICU patients, we applied the EPIC III protocol to estimate the prevalence of community and hospital-associated infections, associated risk factors and distribution of antimicrobial use in the ICUs of the Intensive and Critical Care Department of the University Hospital of Turin. We also evaluated the effectiveness of this data collection protocol as an active surveillance tool.

2. Materials and Methods

2.1. Study Design

This is a 24-h prospective observational point prevalence study, with repeated observations every 2 months. Surveillance was carried out in all medical/surgical ICUs of the Department of Anesthesia and Resuscitation of the Città della Salute e della Scienza Hospital of Turin for a total of 8 ICUs and 72 ICU beds.

The study was approved by the local ethics committee (prot. No.0000255), and informed consent was obtained from each patient enrolled.

The overall duration of the study was 1 year; each observation lasted 24 h, and the follow-up for the outcome was performed at 60 days, regardless of the patient location. Six observations were performed throughout the year, evenly distributed over 12 months. Data were recorded for all patients present or admitted to ICU during the 24-h periods of study, from 1 December 2017, 08:00 to 2 December 2018, 07:59.

All patients hospitalized or admitted to ICU on one of the days of the study were involved, with no exclusion criteria, except for the absence of informed consent.

2.2. Study Context

All ICUs were able to perform blood cultures or qualitative respiratory cultures. Intermittent and continuous renal replacement therapies, high nasal oxygen flow, echocardiography and invasive monitoring were available in all units and extracorporeal membrane oxygenation (ECMO) in two units. An infectious disease specialist or clinical microbiologist was available 12 h a day, 5 days a week, and on-call during nights and weekends. Therapeutic drug monitoring was available for vancomycin, voriconazole, aminoglycosides and beta-lactams.

2.3. Data Collection

Data was collected using the case report form (CRF; see Supplementary Materials) used in EPIC III, investigating presence of infection (up to a maximum of four per patient).

2.4. Operative Definitions

European Centre for Disease Prevention and Control (ECDC) case definitions were applied for infection surveillance [21]. Sepsis and septic shock were defined according to the Third International Consensus Definitions [23]. Multi-drug resistant organisms were defined according to ECDC 2012 definitions [24].

In case of infection, clinicians were asked to classify the mode of acquisition as certainly/possibly/probably and community-acquired/hospital-acquired/ICU-acquired [9].

Infections occurring at least 48 h after hospital admission were defined as 'hospital-acquired'. Infections occurring at least 24 h after ICU admission were defined as 'ICU acquired'. All other infections were defined as 'community-acquired'.

Antimicrobial prophylaxis (not previously defined in the EPIC protocol) was clinically defined as the use of an antimicrobial to prevent the occurrence of an infection, both in medical or surgical contexts.

2.5. Outcomes

Primary outcomes were hospital and 60-days all causes of death. Secondary outcomes were ICU and hospital length of stay (LoS).

2.6. Statistical Analysis

Continuous data are reported as mean and standard deviation (SD) or median and interquartile range (IQR) as appropriate; categorical data are reported as number and percentage. For continuous variables, a comparison between two groups was performed using the unpaired student's t-test or Wilcoxon–Mann–Whitney test depending on type of distribution; for categorical variables, Chi-square test or Fisher's exact test was used as appropriate. Comparison of continuous variables between more than two groups was conducted using Kruskal–Wallis test.

A multivariable logistic regression model was performed using infection as dependent variable and choosing the following covariates resulting significant in the univariate analysis: reason for admission, cardiovascular disease, sex, age, invasive ventilation, vasopressors, central venous access, dialysis and Chronic Obstructive Pulmonary Disease (COPD).

To evaluate possible risk factors for death (60 days mortality), demographic and clinical characteristics associated with mortality were selected as covariates to compete in a multivariable logistic regression model with backward selection.

Results were expressed by calculating the Odd Ratio (OR) and a 95% confidence interval.

All statistical tests were two-sided. p values of 0.05 or less were considered statistically significant and were conducted using the SAS ver. 9.4 (SAS Institute, Cary, NC, USA) and SPSS ver. 26.0 (IBM Corp., Armonk, NY, USA).

3. Results

A total of 435 patients were included in the six study days: 405 adults (mean age 61 years, Standard Deviation (SD) 15, range 18–87) and 30 pediatric patients (mean age

4 years, Standard Deviation (SD) 5, range 0–17). Demographic and general patient data are summarized in Table 1. Informed consent was not collected in less than 5% of patients.

Table 1. Characteristics of patients according to the presence of infection.

		All Patients (n = 435)	Infection		p Value
			No (n = 251)	Yes (n = 184)	
Age, year, mean (SD)		57.5 (20.6)	58 (21.2)	57 (19.7)	0.4069
Male, n (%)		261 (60.0)	141 (56.2)	120 (65.2)	0.0572
ICU, n (%)	General	186 (42.8)	108 (43.0)	78 (42.4)	0.9465
	Specialist	219 (50.3)	125 (49.8)	94 (51.1)	
	Pediatric	30 (6.9)	18 (7.2)	12 (6.5)	
Type of admission, n (%)	Medical	120 (27.6)	46 (18.3)	74 (40.2)	<0.001 *
	Elective surgery	158 (36.3)	114 (45.4)	44 (23.9)	
	Emergency surgery	105 (24.1)	59 (23.5)	46 (25.0)	
	Trauma	52 (12.0)	32 (12.7)	20 (10.9)	
Reason for admission, n (%)	Respiratory	57 (13.1)	13 (5.2)	44 (23.9)	<0.001
	Cardiovascular	55 (12.6)	19 (7.6)	36 (19.6)	
	Neurological	80 (18.4)	46 (18.3)	34 (18.5)	
	Trauma	57 (13.1)	32 (12.7)	25 (13.6)	
	Surveillance	154 (35.4)	125 (49.8)	29 (15.8)	
	Other	32 (7.4)	16 (6.4)	16 (8.7)	
Comorbidities, yes, n (%)		274 (63.0)	159 (63.3)	115 (62.5)	0.8566
Comorbidities, n (%)	Solid cancer	100 (23.0)	68 (15.6)	32 (7.4)	0.0175 *
	Hematologic cancer	7 (1.6)	1 (0.4)	6 (3.3)	0.0452 *
	Diabetes Mellitus	64 (14.7)	42 (16.7)	22 (12.0)	0.1647
	COPD	54 12.4)	21 (8.4)	33 (17.9)	0.0028 *
	Heart Failure, NYHA III/IV	66 (15.2)	36 (14.6)	30 (16.3)	0.5731
	Previous cardiac disease	73 (16.8)	40 (15.9)	33 (17.9)	0.5816
	Chronic kidney failure	55 (12.6)	29 (11.6)	26 (14.1)	0.4244
	Immunosuppression	38 (8.7)	25 (10.0)	13 (7.1)	0.2908
	Solid organ transplant	39 (9.0)	26 (10.4)	13 (7.1)	0.2349
SOFA, mean (SD) [a]		5.5 (4.1)	4.0 (3.2)	7.4 (4.5)	<0.001 *
Invasive ventilation, n (%)		217 (49.9)	96 (38.2)	121 (65.8)	<0.001*
Non-invasive ventilation, n (%)		35 (8.0)	21 (8.5)	14 (7.7)	0.7741
Tracheostomy, n (%)		114 (26.2)	51 (20.6)	63 (34.2)	0.0014 *
Vasopressor use, yes, n (%)		114 (26.2)	50 (19.9)	64 (34.8)	<0.001*
CVC, n (%)		372 (85.5)	206 (83.4)	166 (90.7)	0.0171 *
Urinary catheter, n (%)		407 (93.6)	234 (94.7)	173 (95.1)	0.7386
Renal replacement therapy, n (%)		39 (9.0)	11 (4.4)	28 (15.2)	<0.001 *
ECMO, n (%)		8 (1.8)	0 (0)	8 (4.4)	<0.001 *
Septic shock, n (%)		69 (15.9)	24 (9.6)	45 (24.5)	<0.001 *
Hyperlactacidemia, n (%)		77 (17.7)	37 (14.7)	40 (21.7)	0.0589
Antibiotic prophylaxis, n (%)		149 (34.3)	147 (58.6)	2 (1.1)	<0.001 *
Gastrointestinal decontamination, n (%) [a]		25 (5.9)	12 (4.9)	13 (7.3)	0.2934
Chlorhexidine, n (%) [a]		175 (41.6)	104 (42.4)	71 (40.3)	0.6651
ICU length of stay, days, median (IQR) [a]		14 (4–36)	4 (1–12)	20 (10–33)	<0.001 *
Hospital length of stay, median (IQR) [a]		29 (15–54)	11 (6–21)	50 (22–65)	<0.001 *
Mortality at 60 days, n (%) [a]		52 (12.9)	19 (7.9)	33 (20.1)	<0.001 *

COPD: Chronic obstructive pulmonary disease; CVC: central venous catheter; ECMO: Extracorporeal membrane oxygenation; ICU: Intensive care unit; IQR: interquartile range; NYHA: New York Heart Association; SD: standard deviation; SOFA: Sequential Organ Failure Assessment score, * Significant at 5% level; [a] Total patients are not 435 because of missing values, Percentages are calculated considering missing values.

Overall, 217 patients (50%) were on mechanical ventilation, 69 (16%) were in septic shock, 39 (9%) were treated with extracorporeal renal replacement and 8 (1.8%) with Extracorporeal Membrane Oxygenation (ECMO), and 114 patients (26%), received vasopressor drugs.

Characteristics of the patients according to the ICU type are shown in the Supplementary Material (Table S1A,B). Outcome data on mortality were present for 403 patients. The overall infected patients, according to clinical definition, were 184, whilst the total of patients with at least one positive isolate was 114.

3.1. *Prevalence of Infections*

The infection section of the CRF was completed for 425 patients (98%). A total of 184 patients (42%) had at least one infection on one of the study days: 126 patients (69%) at one site, 48 patients (26%) at two sites and 58 (32%) in more than two sites.

The proportion of infected patients was 42%, 43% and 40% in general, specialist and pediatric ICUs respectively (Table 1).

Among infected patients (184), 114 (62%) had at least one positive isolate at microbiological culture. ICU-acquired infections were the most common (117 patients—64%), followed by hospital or healthcare-associated infections (41 patients—22%) and community-acquired (36 patients—20%). Data regarding infection acquisition are reported in Table 2.

Table 2. Infection characteristics according to mode of acquisition and microbiological isolates (note: 184 infected patients, 114 culture-positive patients).

			Mode of Acquisition		
		Infected Patients (n = 184)	**Community-Acquired (n = 36)**	**Hospital-Acquired/Health Care-Associated (n = 41)**	**ICU-Acquired (n = 117)**
Evidence of infection, n (%)	Certain	108 (58.7)	25 (69.4)	22 (53.7)	74 (63.2)
	Probable	44 (23.9)	10 (27.8)	8 (19.5)	30 (25.6)
	Feasible	52 (28.3)	5 (13.9)	20 (48.8)	32 (27.4)
Site of infection, n (%)	Respiratory system	114 (62.0)	23 (63.9)	25 (61.0)	77 (65.8)
	Abdomen	21 (11.4)	3 (8.3)	9 (22.0)	10 (8.5)
	Circulation	69 (37.5)	11 (30.6)	12 (29.3)	56 (47.9)
	Kidney/genitourinary	17 (9.2)	2 (5.6)	3 (7.3)	14 (12.0)
	Others	26 (14.1)	6 (16.7)	6 (14.6)	14 (12.0)
		Colture-Positive Patients (n = 114)	**Community-Acquired (n = 16)**	**Hospital-Acquired/Health Care-Associated (n = 23)**	**ICU-Acquired (n = 85)**
Positive isolates, n (%)	Gram-positive	34 (29.8)	6 (37.5)	8 (34.8)	24 (28.2)
	Gram-positive MS	19 (16.7)	5 (31.3)	5 (21.7)	12 (14.1)
	Gram-positive MDR	17 (14.9)	1 (6.3)	5 (21.7)	14 (16.5)
	Gram-negative	98 (86.0)	10 (62.5)	17 (73.9)	78 (91.8)
	Gram-negative MS	69 (60.5)	9 (56.3)	9 (39.1)	56 (65.9)
	Gram-negative MDR	47 (41.2)	2 (12.5)	10 (43.5)	39 (45.9)
	All MDR bacteria	59 (51.8)	3 (18.8)	14 (60.9)	48 (56.5)
	Fungi	19 (16.7)	5 (31.3)	3 (13.0)	14 (16.5)
	Viruses	8 (7.0)	5 (31.3)	1 (4.3)	4 (4.7)
	Klebsiella	40 (35.1)	3 (18.8)	10 (43.5)	30 (35.3)
	Pseudomonas	30 (26.3)	1 (6.3)	2 (8.7)	28 (32.9)
	Acinetobacter	16 (14.0)	0 (0)	2 (8.7)	15 (17.6)
	Bacteria resistant to Carbapenems	36 (31.6)	1 (6.3)	8 (34.8)	30 (35.3)

ICU: intensive care unit; MDR multi-drug resistant; MS: multi-sensitive. Percentages can exceed 100% because patients could have more than one infection.

Infection characteristics according to mortality (403 patients, lacking mortality data of 32 patients) are shown in Table 3.

Table 3. Infection characteristics according to mortality (note: total number of patients is 403, as 32 patients' outcome data were missing).

		All Patients (*n* = 403)	Mortality at 60 Days		*p* Value
			Alive (*n* = 351)	Dead (*n* = 52)	
Antibiotic prophylaxis, *n* (%)		141 (35.2)	131 (37.4)	10 (19.6)	0.0107 *
Positive isolates, *n* (%)	Gram-positive	33 (8.2)	30 (8.5)	3 (5.8)	0.7852
	Gram-positive MS	19 (4.7)	18 (5.1)	1 (1.9)	0.4891
	Gram-positive MDR	16 (4.0)	14 (4.0)	2 (3.8)	1.0000
	Gram-negative	87 (21.6)	76 (21.7)	11 (21.2)	0.9350
	Gram-negative MS	60 (14.9)	52 (14.8)	8 (15.4)	0.9142
	Gram-negative MDR	42 (10.4)	37 (10.5)	5 (9.6)	0.8384
	All MDR bacteria	54 (13.4)	47 (13.4)	7 (13.5)	0.9888
	Fungi	16 (4.0)	9 (2.6)	7 (13.5)	0.0018 *
	Viruses	6 (1.5)	5 (1.4)	1 (1.9)	0.5659
	Klebsiella	36 (8.9)	35 (10.0)	1 (1.9)	0.0664
	Pseudomonas	28 (6.9)	25 (7.1)	3 (5.8)	1.0000
	Acinetobacter	15 (3.7)	13 (3.7)	2 (3.8)	1.0000
	Bacteria resistant to Carbapenems	32 (7.9)	28 (8.0)	4 (7.7)	1.0000
Site of infection, *n* (%)	Respiratory system	102 (25.3)	80 (22.8)	22 (42.3)	0.0025 *
	Abdomen	16 (4.0)	13 (3.7)	3 (5.8)	0.4460
	Circulation	56 (13.9)	40 (11.4)	16 (30.8)	0.0002 *
	Kidney/genitourinary	16 (4.0)	13 (3.7)	3 (5.8)	0.4460
	Others	24 (6.0)	21 (6.0)	3 (5.8)	1.0000
Acquisition mode, *n* (%)	Community-acquired	30 (7.4)	20 (5.7)	10 (19.2)	0.0022 *
	Hospital-acquired /Health Care-associated	36 (8.9)	27 (7.7)	9 (17.3)	0.0344 *
	ICU-acquired	106 (26.3)	87 (24.8)	19 (36.5)	0.0724

MDR: multi-drug resistant; MS: multi-sensitive; ICU: intensive care unit. * Significant at 5% level.

Considering patients with at least one positive microbiological culture (total = 114), Gram-positive bacteria were isolated in 34 patients (30%); Gram-negative bacteria were isolated in 98 (86%); 59 patients (52%) presented one or multiple multidrug-resistant (MDR) bacteria, as follows: gram-negative MDR in 47 patients (41%); gram-positive MDR in 17 patients (15%). Methicillin-resistant Staphylococcus aureus (MRSA) was isolated in 10 patients (8.8%). No cases of C. difficile (CD) have been reported. Other isolates were fungi (19 patients [17%]), viruses (8 [7%]) and anaerobes (1 [1%]). *Klebsiella* spp. was isolated in 40 patients (35%), *Pseudomonas* spp. in 30 (26%) and *Acinetobacter* spp. in 16 (14%); the total of patients with an infection caused by Carbapenem-resistant bacteria was 36 (32%). Details on sites of infection and isolated microorganisms are shown in Figure 1.

A total of 256 infections were clinically diagnosed in 184 patients overall; these were considered definite, probable or possible in 108 (59%), 44 (24%) and 52 (28%) patients, respectively.

Considering the overall number of isolates (total = 170), MDR or resistance to carbapenems were 49% and 21%, respectively, of the total of isolates.

The multivariate analysis carried out to evaluate the impact of different factors on infections evidenced that invasive ventilation, renal replacement therapy and COPD as comorbidity prior to hospitalization are all factors independently associated with an increased risk of developing an infection (Table 4A,B).

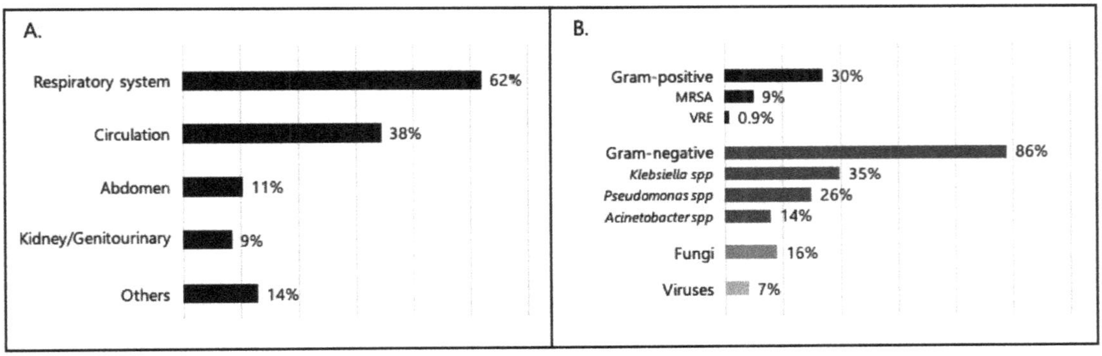

Figure 1. Site of infection and isolated microorganism. (**A**). Infection sites in infected patients ($N = 184$). (**B**). Isolated microorganisms in culture-positive patients ($N = 114$). Percentages can exceed 100% because patients could have more than one infection.

Table 4. (**A**) Univariate and multivariable logistic regression analysis with infection as the dependent variable. (**B**) Univariate and multivariable logistic regression analysis with mortality at 60 days as the dependent variable.

(A)			
		Univariate	**Multivariate**
Variable		**OR (95% CI)**	**OR (95% CI)**
Age		1.00 (0.99–1.01)	1.00 (0.99–1.01)
Gender	Male	1 (reference)	1 (reference)
	Female	0.69 (0.47–1.02)	0.92 (0.57–1.48))
Reason for admission	Respiratory	1 (reference)	1 (reference)
	Cardiovascular	0.56 (0.24–1.29)	0.37 (0.15–0.92)
	Neurological	0.22 (0.10–0.47)	0.23 (0.10–0.53)
	Trauma	0.23 (0.10–0.52)	0.29 (0.12–0.68)
	Surveillance	0.07 (0.03–0.15)	0.07 (0.03–0.15)
	Other	0.30 (0.12–0.75)	0.25 (0.09–0.69)
Invasive ventilation		3.13 (2.11–4.66)	2.14 (1.29–3.53)
Vasopressor use		2.19 (1.42–3.38)	1.53 (0.86–2.73)
CVC		1.97 (1.10–3.54)	1.37 (0.68–2.74)
Renal replacement therapy		3.90 (1.89–8.06)	2.78 (1.30–5.96)
COPD		2.38 (1.33–4.28)	2.15 (1.06–4.35)
(B)			
Variable		**OR (95% CI)**	**OR (95% CI)**
Age		1.04 (1.02–1.07)	1.05 (1.02–1.08)
Gender	Male	1 (reference)	1 (reference)
	Female	1.20 (0.66–2.16)	2.20 (1.07–4.53)

Table 4. *Cont.*

Source of admission	Operating room/Surgical department	1 (reference)	1 (reference)
	Emergency department	1.13 (0.51–2.48)	1.03 (0.38–2.78)
	Medical department	3.56 (1.53–8.26)	3.69 (1.39–9.78)
	Other hospital	0.86 (0.27–2.69)	0.59 (0.15–2.35)
	Other ICUs	2.01 (0.76–5.29)	3.86 (1.16–12.84)
Comorbidities		11.53 (3.52–37.73)	12.77 (2.91–56.02)
Invasive ventilation		4.71 (2.34–9.48)	4.22 (1.91–9.30)
Site of infection	Circulation	3.56 (1.81–7.00)	3.43 (1.48–7.97)
Acquisition mode	Community-acquired	4.04 (1.77–9.22)	9.90 (3.07–31.92)

CI: confidence interval; COPD: Chronic obstructive pulmonary disease; CVC: central venous catheter; OR: odds ratio. ICU: intensive care unit.

3.2. Antibiotic Therapy

On the six study days, 311 patients (72%) were receiving at least one antibiotic: 149 patients (48%) for medical or surgical prophylaxis and 162 (52%) for treatment. Prophylaxis was performed with one antibiotic in 101 patients (68%) and with two or more antibiotics in 48 patients (32%). Cefazolin was the most used prophylactic antibiotic (42 patients—28%), followed by amoxicillin–clavulanate (28 patients—19%) and piperacillin–tazobactam (27 patients—18%).

Antibiotic therapy was carried out with one antibiotic in 44 cases (27%), with two antibiotics in 57 cases (35%) and with three to five antibiotics in 61 cases (37%). The most frequently used molecules were meropenem (39 patients—24%), piperacillin–tazobactam (38 patients—23%) and levofloxacin (27 patients—17%). Meropenem, piperacillin–tazobactam were the most used antibiotics in patients with hospital-acquired infection (34% and 29% respectively) and ICU-acquired infection (20% and 15% respectively). Piperacillin-tazobactam, ceftriaxone and metronidazole were the most used antibiotics in patients with community-acquired infection.

3.3. Clinical Outcomes

Mortality of the cohort included in the present study was 13% with a statistically significant difference between patients without and with infection (8% vs. 20%; $p < 0.001$). Median LoS in ICU and hospital was 14 (IQR 4–36) and 29 (IQR 15–54) days, respectively, and was significantly different in patients without and with infection: 4 (1–12) vs. 20 (13–33) days ($p < 0.001$) and 11 (6–21) vs. 50 (22–65) days ($p < 0.001$), as shown in Table 5.

Table 5. Characteristics of patients according to mortality (note: total number of patients is 403, as in 32 patients outcome data were missing).

		All Patients (n = 403)	Mortality at 60 Days		p Value
			Alive (n = 351)	Dead (n = 52)	
Age, year, mean (SD)		57.5 (20.6)	56.5 (22.9)	66.6 (15.0)	<0.001 *
Male, n (%)		236 (58.6)	208 (59.3)	28 (53.8)	0.4596
ICU, n (%)	General	173 (42.9)	146 (41.6)	27 (51.9)	<0.001 *
	Specialist	203 (50.4)	180 (51.3)	23 (44.2)	
	Pediatric	27 (6.7)	25 (7.1)	11 (3.8)	

Table 5. *Cont.*

		All Patients (n = 403)	Mortality at 60 Days		p Value
			Alive (n = 351)	Dead (n = 52)	
Type of admission, n (%)	Medical	109 (27.0)	87 (24.8)	22 (42.3)	0.0122 *
	Surgical election	151 (37.5)	135 (38.5)	16 (30.8)	
	Surgical emergency	95 (23.6)	82 (23.4)	13 (25.0)	
	Trauma	48 (11.9)	47 (13.4)	1 (21.9)	
Reason for admission, n (%)	Respiratory	52 (13.0)	41 (11.7)	11 (21.2)	<0.001 *
	Cardiovascular	50 (12.4)	36 (10.3)	14 (26.9)	
	Neurological	72 (17.9)	64 (18.2)	8 (15.4)	
	Trauma	53 (13.2)	52 (14.8)	1 (1.9)	
	Surveillance	147 (36.2)	134 (37.8)	13 (25.0)	
	Other	29 (7.2)	24 (6.8)	5 (17.2)	
Comorbidities, yes, n (%)		252 (62.5)	204 (58.1)	48 (92.3)	<0.001 *
Comorbidities, n (%)	Solid cancer	94 (23.3)	77 (19.1)	17 (4.2)	0.0870
	Hematologic cancer	6 (1.5)	3 (0.9)	3 (5.8)	0.0306 *
	Diabetes Mellitus	60 (14.9)	50 (14.2)	10 (19.2)	0.3459
	COPD	50 (12.4)	35 (10.0)	15 (28.8)	<0.001 *
	Heart Failure, NYHA III/IV	59 (14.6)	46 (13.1)	13 (25.0)	0.0236 *
	Previous cardiac disease	68 (16.9)	47 (13.4)	21 (40.4)	<0.001 *
	Chronic kidney failure	48 (11.9)	36 (10.3)	12 (23.1)	0.0077 *
	Immunosuppression	36 (8.9)	30 (8.5)	6 (11.5)	0.4405
	Solid-organ transplant	36 (8.9)	31 (8.8)	5 (9.6)	0.7965
SOFA, mean (SD) [a]		5.5 (4.1)	4.5 (3.6)	9.6 (4.1)	<0.001*
Invasive ventilation, n (%)		194 (48.1)	153 (43.6)	41 (78.8)	<0.001 *
Non-invasive ventilation, n (%)		33 (8.3)	28 (8.1)	5 (9.6)	0.5971
Tracheostomy, n (%)		101 (25.3)	87 (25.0)	14 (26.9)	0.7401
Vasopressor use, yes, n (%)		101 (25.1)	75 (21.4)	26 (50.0)	<0.001 *
CVC, n (%)		343 (86.0)	294 (84.7)	49 (94.2)	0.0478 *
Urinary catheter, n (%)		376 (94.7)	325 (94.2)	51 (98.1)	0.2300
Renal replacement therapy, n (%)		36 (8.9)	23 (6.6)	13 (25.0)	<0.001 *
ECMO, n (%)		7 (1.8)	6 (1.7)	1 (1.9)	1.0000
Septic shock, n (%)		58 (14.4)	42 (12.0)	16 (30.8)	<0.001 *
Hyperlactacidemia, n (%)		64 (15.9)	47 (13.4)	17 (32.7)	<0.001 *
ICU length of stay, days, median (IQR) [a]		14 (4–35)	14 (3–34)	14 (8–45)	0.2494
Hospital length of stay, median (IQR) [a]		29 (16–54)	28 (16–52)	39 (14–68)	0.4315

COPD: Chronic obstructive pulmonary disease; CVC: central venous catheter; ECMO: Extracorporeal membrane oxygenation; ICU: Intensive care unit; IQR: interquartile range; NYHA: New York Heart Association; SD: standard deviation; SOFA: Sequential Organ Failure Assessment score. * Significant at 5% level; [a] Total patients are not 435 because of missing values. Percentages are calculated considering missing values.

The multivariate analysis carried out to evaluate the impact of different factors on mortality at 60 days evidenced that invasive ventilation, confirmed bloodstream infection, community-acquired infection and presence of at least one comorbid condition were independently associated with a higher risk of mortality (Table 4).

4. Discussion

Data collected in this six-days point prevalence study, bi-monthly repeated in eight ICUs of a university hospital in Turin (Italy) between 2017 and 2018, evidenced an overall prevalence of infection of 42%. This estimate is lower than the rate found by the international EPIC III study (54%), which already showed an upward trend compared to previous EPIC studies (45% for EPIC I in 1992 [25] and 51% for EPIC II in 2007 [26]).

In our cohort, the proportion of patients with ICU-acquired infection was higher compared to the EPIC III study (26.3% vs. 21.6%). When hospital-acquired infections are also considered, we found an additional 8.9% (compared to 34.5% in the EPIC III cohort). Overall, ICU-acquired infections accounted for 64% of infections, followed by hospital-acquired (22%) and community-acquired (20%) infections, considering that each patient may have developed more than one infection type.

It is well known that HAIs represent a major patient safety issue as well as a significant economic burden, being frequently characterized by antimicrobial resistance. Among European countries, Italy is one of those where antibiotic use and prevalence of antimicrobial resistance in both the community and hospital settings are highest [14,27,28]. Even if ICU is the clinical setting in which HAI prevalence is highest, with data ranging between 19.5% in Europe [19], and 35–36.8% [29,30] in North Italy, there is a lack of specific data based on the ECDC surveillance model and repeated over time. We therefore consider the model proposed here particularly interesting for its ability to evaluate the evolution over time in the specific ecological context of reference.

Our data confirm the role that infections play in mortality. Although hospital mortality was, overall, low (12.9%) and different according to the type of ICUs (from 47.6 to 2.9%—Supplementary Materials, Table S1A,B), the impact of infection on mortality seems notable (20.1% vs. 7.9%, $p < 0.001$).

Infections seem to obviously affect even the length of ICU and hospital stay (4 (1–12) vs. 20 (13–33) days ($p < 0.001$) and 11 (6–21) vs. 50 (22–65) days ($p < 0.001$), respectively). Mechanical ventilation, the presence of medical devices such as a central venous catheter, renal replacement therapy, ECMO and tracheostomy are all factors independently associated with an increased infections risk even if, at multivariate analysis, only invasive ventilation, renal replacement therapy and COPD were independently associated with a higher risk of infection. In line with EPIC III results, older age and the presence of at least one comorbidity were all factors independently associated with a higher risk of death in our cohort. Interestingly, multivariate analysis found that also male gender, admission from the medical department or referral from other ICUs, invasive ventilation, confirmed bloodstream infection and community as a source of infection are factors associated with an increased risk of death.

Regarding microbiological isolation, considering patients with at least one positive microbiological culture, in line with EPIC III data and international literature [3,6,8], Gram-negative microorganisms were more frequently identified than gram-positive microorganisms (86% vs. 30%). 41% of patients had an infection sustained by Gram-negative MDR bacteria (12), *Klebsiella* spp., *Pseudomonas* spp. and *Acinetobacter* spp. the most represented (35%, 26% and 14% of microbiological isolates, respectively). The high proportion of carbapenem-resistant organisms (21% of the total isolates) confirmed the increasing trend already emerged from the ECDC and EARS-Net data relating to Italy [19,27,31]. Infections due to Gram-negative pathogens, and especially to MDR bacteria, are more frequent considering hospital-associated and ICU-associated infections. In fact, Gram-negative bacteria were isolated in 63%, 74% and 92% of patients with culture-positive infection acquired in community, hospital and ICU, respectively. Gram-negative MDR bacteria were responsible for infection in 12%, 43% and 46% of patients with culture-positive infection acquired in community, hospital and ICU, respectively (Table 2).

Probably due to the limited sample size, no microorganism was identified as independently and significantly associated with higher mortality risk. This also applies to carbapenem-resistant *Klebsiella* and *Acinetobacter* species, which are listed among the most critical antibiotic-resistant pathogens by the World Health Organization and to which a particular role in increasing the risk of death is universally attributed [31,32].

In line with the EPIC III study, even in our cohort, we found that 72% of patients received at least one systemic antimicrobial agent for prophylactic or therapeutic purposes (34.5% and 37.5% of total patients, respectively). In a significant percentage of cases, combination choices were made for both prophylaxis (32%) and therapy (72%). These data reflect an increasingly widespread but dangerous practice which, instead, deserves close monitoring, due to the high risk of developing resistance, particularly in the context of critically ill patients [33–35]. Given the rarity of cases in which the combined use of antibiotics allows a synergistic effect of antibiotics, the use of combined therapy with the aim of increasing the spectrum of action should be reserved for specific cases, such as multidrug-resistant pathogens treatment, to be closely monitored for prompt de-escalation [36–38].

Equally worthy of particular attention is the frequent use of beta-lactams in combination for prophylactic (37% of cases) instead of the therapeutic purpose of carbapenems (30% of cases) and quinolones (24%) for therapeutic purposed. Both of these practices should be carefully monitored given the ECDC, which seem to suggest, in Europe and in particular in Italy, the presence of a high resistance rate [19,27].

A final aspect of our analysis of particular interest is that our data refer to 8 different ICUs, admitting, with different modalities (emergency/scheduled), patients with different characteristics and severity (Supplementary Materials, Table S1A,B). This obviously reflects the 60-day mortality rate, ICU and hospital LoS, and infections, since different case mixes and risk factors have a different impact on the clinical course of patients and the approach to antibiotic therapy applied by clinicians.

For this reason, on one hand, it is essential to repeat the comparison over time of the data obtained in every single ICU, taking into account the patient selection bias. On the other hand, since the ICUs included in the study are located in a similar context (i.e., the same hospital) characterized by methods for the diagnosis of infection, microbiology ecology and similar infection control and antimicrobial stewardship policies, the repeated serial comparison allows effective monitoring of the effectiveness of the corrective measured implemented over time.

Those two aspects—center-specific peculiarities on one side, homogeneity of microbiology ecology and local policies on the other side—should be considered together when planning and interpreting the results of present and future surveillance programs or interventions.

We believe that the proposal to repeatedly apply a prevalence survey tool may be particularly effective in allowing repeated comparison over time in the same (or at least similar) setting, in order to identify the emergence of new criticalities or to effectively monitor the introduction of possible corrective measures.

Limitations

This study has limitations. First, our study collected data from eight different ICUs in a large acute-care hospital. Results are, hence, not generalizable to smaller hospitals, since infection prevalence may vary greatly with hospital beds number and case mix.

Second, to preserve the easy-to-use format of the EPIC III model [9], some aspects of infections were not approached such as timing and differentiation between acute and resolution phases. Furthermore, no data on colonization and general ICU approach to surveillance cultures were collected. Finally, no follow-up data were collected with the exception of 60 days mortality.

5. Conclusions

In this study, we highlighted a relatively high prevalence of infections and antimicrobial use and brought out specific critical issues relating to the different specialist ICU contexts. Considering that these aspects require continuous reassessment over time to evaluate the effects of all corrective actions implemented, we believe the repeated punctual prevalence survey represents a quick, easily repeatable, and economical method to accomplish infections and antimicrobial use surveillance in ICUs, pointing out the priorities that need improvement actions and providing feedback to health care professionals. The use of the ECDC definitions and the EPIC III protocol, known and used all over the world, is strategic to allow comparisons with national and international contexts. In addition, this surveillance might be easily repeated in the same facility, allowing monitoring of local microbiological ecology and antimicrobial use during the time to promptly identify main problematic factors and plan for specific improvement actions.

Further studies are needed to better clarify the role of prevalence investigations in infectious surveillance and their role in antimicrobial stewardship and to identify the most effective interventions to optimize antimicrobial management, especially in intensive care.

Supplementary Materials: The following supporting information can be downloaded at: https://www.mdpi.com/article/10.3390/jcm11092482/s1. Case Report Form (CRF); Table S1. (A) Characteristics of patients according to the ICU type. (B) Characteristics of infection according to the ICU type.

Author Contributions: Conceptualization, G.M. and L.B.; methodology, G.M., L.B., G.S. and C.F.; software, C.F.; validation and formal analysis, C.F. and G.C.; investigation, G.M., G.S., S.C. and G.C.; resources, G.M., G.S., A.C., R.U. and L.B.; data curation, G.M., G.S., S.B., M.S., T.V.V. and A.C.; writing—original draft preparation, G.M. and G.C.; writing—review and editing, G.S., A.C., R.U., L.B., S.C. and F.G.D.R.; supervision, L.B. and F.G.D.R. All authors have read and agreed to the published version of the manuscript.

Funding: This research received no external funding.

Institutional Review Board Statement: The study was conducted according to the guidelines of the Declaration of Helsinki, and approved by the Ethics Committee of Città della Salute e della Scienza Hospital (protocol code 0000255 and 02012018).

Informed Consent Statement: Informed consent was obtained from all subjects involved in the study.

Data Availability Statement: Data available on reasonable request from the authors.

Acknowledgments: The Authors thank all physicians, nurses and collaborators involved in the daily care of patients in each ICU of our Department, who made this study possible.

Conflicts of Interest: The authors declare no conflict of interest influencing the representation or interpretation of reported research results.

References

1. Sakr, Y.; Jaschinski, U.; Wittebole, X.; Szakmany, T.; Lipman, J.; Ñamendys-Silva, S.A.; Martin-Loeches, I.; Leone, M.; Lupu, M.-N.; Vincent, J.-L.; et al. Sepsis in Intensive Care Unit Patients: Worldwide Data from the Intensive Care over Nations Audit. *Open Forum Infect. Dis.* **2018**, *5*, ofy313. [CrossRef] [PubMed]
2. SepNet Critical Care Trials Group. Incidence of severe sepsis and septic shock in German intensive care units: The prospective, multicentre INSEP study. *Intensive Care Med.* **2016**, *42*, 1980–1989. [CrossRef] [PubMed]
3. Baykara, N.; Sepsis Study Group; Akalın, H.; Arslantaş, M.K.; Hancı, V.; Çağlayan, Ç.; Kahveci, F.; Demirağ, K.; Baydemir, C.; Ünal, N. Epidemiology of sepsis in intensive care units in Turkey: A multicenter, point-prevalence study. *Crit. Care* **2018**, *22*, 93. [CrossRef] [PubMed]
4. Zhou, J.; Qian, C.; Zhao, M.; Yu, X.; Kang, Y.; Ma, X.; Ai, Y.; Xu, Y.; Liu, D.; An, Y.; et al. Epidemiology and outcome of severe sepsis and septic shock in intensive care units in mainland China. *PLoS ONE* **2014**, *9*, e107181. [CrossRef] [PubMed]
5. Silva, E.; Dalfior, L., Jr.; Fernandes Hda, S.; Moreno, R.; Vincent, J.L. Prevalence and outcomes of infections in Brazilian ICUs: A subanalysis of EPIC II study. Prevalência e desfechos clínicos de infecções em UTIs brasileiras: Subanálise do estudo EPIC II. *Rev. Bras. Ter. Intensiva* **2012**, *24*, 143–150. [CrossRef] [PubMed]
6. Agodi, A.; Barchitta, M.; Auxilia, F. Epidemiology of intensive care unit-acquired sepsis in Italy: Results of the SPIN-UTI network. *Ann. Ig.* **2018**, *30* (Suppl. 2), 15–21. [CrossRef]
7. Migliara, G.; Di Paolo, C.; Barbato, D. Multimodal surveillance of healthcare associated infections in an intensive care unit of a large teaching hospital. *Ann. Ig.* **2019**, *31*, 399–413. [CrossRef]
8. Reinhart, K.; Daniels, R.; Kissoon, N.; Machado, F.R.; Schachter, R.D.; Finfer, S. Recognizing Sepsis as a Global Health Priority—A WHO Resolution. *N. Engl. J. Med.* **2017**, *377*, 414–417. [CrossRef]
9. Vincent, J.-L.; Sakr, Y.; Singer, M.; Martin-Loeches, I.; Machado, F.R.; Marshall, J.C.; Finfer, S.; Pelosi, P.; Brazzi, L.; Aditianingsih, D.; et al. Prevalence and Outcomes of Infection Among Patients in Intensive Care Units in 2017. *JAMA* **2020**, *323*, 1478–1487. [CrossRef]
10. Li, Z.-J.; Wang, K.-W.; Liu, B.; Zang, F.; Zhang, Y.; Zhang, W.-H.; Zhou, S.-M.; Zhang, Y.-X. The Distribution and Source of MRDOs Infection: A Retrospective Study in 8 ICUs, 2013–2019. *Infect. Drug Resist.* **2021**, *14*, 4983–4991. [CrossRef]
11. Saito, H.; Kilpatrick, C.; Pittet, D. The 2018 World Health Organization SAVE LIVES: Clean Your Hands Campaign targets sepsis in health care. *Intensive Care Med.* **2018**, *44*, 499–501. [CrossRef] [PubMed]

12. Markwart, R.; Saito, H.; Harder, T.; Tomczyk, S.; Cassini, A.; Fleischmann-Struzek, C.; Reichert, F.; Eckmanns, T.; Allegranzi, B. Epidemiology and burden of sepsis acquired in hospitals and intensive care units: A systematic review and meta-analysis. *Intensive Care Med.* **2020**, *46*, 1536–1551. [CrossRef] [PubMed]
13. World Health Organization. *Report on the Burden of Endemic Health Care-Associated Infection Worldwide*; World Health Organization: Geneva, Switzerland, 2011; Available online: https://apps.who.int/iris/bitstream/handle/10665/80135/9789241501507_eng.pdf (accessed on 16 March 2022).
14. Suetens, C.; Latour, K.; Kärki, T.; Ricchizzi, E.; Kinross, P.; Moro, M.L.; Jans, B.; Hopkins, S.; Hansen, S.; Lyytikäinen, O.; et al. Prevalence of healthcare-associated infections, estimated incidence and composite antimicrobial resistance index in acute care hospitals and long-term care facilities: Results from two European point prevalence surveys, 2016 to 2017. *Euro Surveill.* **2018**, *23*, 1800516. [CrossRef] [PubMed]
15. Schreiber, P.W.; Sax, H.; Wolfensberger, A.; Clack, L.; Kuster, S.P. The preventable proportion of healthcare-associated infections 2005-2016: Systematic review and meta-analysis. *Infect. Control Hosp. Epidemiol.* **2018**, *39*, 1277–1295. [CrossRef] [PubMed]
16. Rudd, K.E.; Johnson, S.C.; Agesa, K.M.; Shackelford, K.A.; Tsoi, D.; Kievlan, D.R.; Colombara, D.V.; Ikuta, K.S.; Kissoon, N.; Finfer, S.; et al. Global, regional, and national sepsis incidence and mortality, 1990–2017: Analysis for the Global Burden of Disease Study. *Lancet* **2020**, *395*, 200–211. [CrossRef]
17. Fleischmann, M.C.; Scherag, A.; Adhikari, N.K.J.; Hartog, C.S.; Tsaganos, T.; Schlattmann, P.; Angus, D.C.; Reinhart, K.; International Forum of Acute Care Trialists. Assessment of Global Incidence and Mortality of Hospital-treated Sepsis. Current Estimates and Limitations. *Am. J. Respir. Crit. Care Med* **2016**, *193*, 259–272. [CrossRef]
18. Finazzi, S.; Paci, G.; Antiga, L.; Brissy, O.; Carrara, G.; Crespi, D.; Csato, G.; Csomos, A.; Duek, O.; Facchinetti, S.; et al. PROSAFE: A European endeavor to improve quality of critical care medicine in seven countries. *Minerva Anestesiol.* **2020**, *86*, 1305–1320. [CrossRef]
19. Weist, K.; Högberg, L.D. ECDC publishes 2015 surveillance data on antimicrobial resistance and antimicrobial consumption in Europe. *Eurosurveillance* **2016**, *21*, 30401. [CrossRef]
20. Serra-Burriel, M.; Campillo-Artero, C.; Agodi, A.; Barchitta, M.; López-Casasnovas, G. Association between antibiotic resistance in intensive care unit (ICU)-acquired infections and excess resource utilization: Evidence from Spain, Italy, and Portugal. *Infect. Control Hosp. Epidemiol.* **2021**. [CrossRef]
21. Plachouras, D.; Lepape, A.; Suetens, C. ECDC definitions and methods for the surveillance of healthcare-associated infections in intensive care units. *Intensive Care Med.* **2018**, *44*, 2216–2218. [CrossRef]
22. Yin, M.; Tambyah, P.A.; Perencevich, E.N. Infection, Antibiotics, and Patient Outcomes in the Intensive Care Unit. *JAMA* **2020**, *323*, 1451–1452. [CrossRef] [PubMed]
23. Singer, M.; Deutschman, C.S.; Seymour, C.W.; Shankar-Hari, M.; Annane, D.; Bauer, M.; Bellomo, R.; Bernard, G.R.; Chiche, J.-D.; Coopersmith, C.M.; et al. The Third International Consensus Definitions for Sepsis and Septic Shock (Sepsis-3). *JAMA* **2016**, *315*, 801–810. [CrossRef] [PubMed]
24. Magiorakos, A.-P.; Srinivasan, A.; Carey, R.B.; Carmeli, Y.; Falagas, M.E.; Giske, C.G.; Harbarth, S.; Hindler, J.F.; Kahlmeter, G.; Olsson-Liljequist, B.; et al. Multidrug-resistant, extensively drug-resistant and pandrug-resistant bacteria: An international expert proposal for interim standard definitions for acquired resistance. *Clin. Microbiol. Infect.* **2012**, *18*, 268–281. [CrossRef] [PubMed]
25. Vincent, J.-L.; Bihari, D.J.; Suter, P.M.; Bruining, H.A.; White, J.; Nicolas-Chanoin, M.-H.; Wolff, M.; Spencer, R.C.; Hemmer, M. The prevalence of nosocomial infection in intensive care units in Europe. Results of the European Prevalence of Infection in Intensive Care (EPIC) Study. EPIC International Advisory Committee. *JAMA* **1995**, *274*, 639–644. [CrossRef] [PubMed]
26. Vincent, J.-L.; Rello, J.; Marshall, J.K.; Silva, E.; Anzueto, A.; Martin, C.D.; Moreno, R.; Lipman, J.; Gomersall, C.; Sakr, Y.; et al. International study of the prevalence and outcomes of infection in intensive care units. *JAMA* **2009**, *302*, 2323–2329. [CrossRef]
27. European Centre for Disease Prevention and Control. Antimicrobial consumption. In *ECDC Annual Epidemiological Report for 2017*; ECDC: Stockholm, Sweden, 2018; Available online: http://ecdc.europa.eu/sites/portal/files/documents/AER_for_2017-antimicrobial-consumption.pdf (accessed on 16 March 2022).
28. Secondo Studio di Prevalenza Italiano Sulle Infezioni Correlate All'assistenza e Sull'Uso di Antibiotici Negli Ospedali per Acuti—Protocollo ECDC. Dipartimento Scienze Della Salute Pubblica e Pediatriche Università di Torino. 2018. Available online: http://www.salute.gov.it/imgs/C_17_pubblicazioni_2791_allegato.pdf (accessed on 16 March 2022).
29. Antonioli, P.; Bolognesi, N.; Valpiani, G.; Morotti, C.; Bernardini, D.; Bravi, F.; Di Ruscio, E.; Stefanati, A.; Gabutti, G. A 2-year point-prevalence surveillance of healthcare-associated infections and antimicrobial use in Ferrara University Hospital, Italy. *BMC Infect. Dis.* **2020**, *20*, 75. [CrossRef]
30. Metsini, A.; Vazquez, M.; Sommerstein, R.; Marschall, J.; Voide, C.; Troillet, N.; Gardiol, C.; Pittet, D.; Zingg, W. Point prevalence of healthcare-associated infections and antibiotic use in three large Swiss acute-care hospitals. *Swiss Med. Wkly.* **2018**, *148*, w14617. [CrossRef]
31. Cassini, A.; Högberg, L.D.; Plachouras, D.; Quattrocchi, A.; Hoxha, A.; Simonsen, G.S.; Colomb-Cotinat, M.; Kretzschmar, M.E.; Devleesschauwer, B.; Cecchini, M.; et al. Attributable deaths and disability-adjusted life-years caused by infections with antibiotic-resistant bacteria in the EU and the European Economic Area in 2015: A population-level modelling analysis. *Lancet Infect. Dis.* **2019**, *19*, 56–66. [CrossRef]

32. Tacconelli, E.; Carrara, E.; Savoldi, A.; Harbarth, S.; Mendelson, M.; Monnet, D.L.; Pulcini, C.; Kahlmeter, G.; Kluytmans, J.; Carmeli, Y.; et al. Discovery, research, and development of new antibiotics: The WHO priority list of antibiotic-resistant bacteria and tuberculosis. *Lancet Infect. Dis.* **2018**, *18*, 318–327. [CrossRef]
33. Montrucchio, G.; Sales, G.; Corcione, S.; De Rosa, F.G.; Brazzi, L. Choosing wisely: What is the actual role of antimicrobial stewardship in Intensive Care Units? *Minerva Anestesiol.* **2019**, *85*, 71–82. [CrossRef]
34. De Rosa, F.G.; Corcione, S.; Montrucchio, G.; Brazzi, L.; Di Perri, G. Antifungal Treatment Strategies in the ICU: Beyond Meta-analysis. *Turk. J. Anaesthesiol. Reanim.* **2016**, *44*, 283–284. [CrossRef] [PubMed]
35. De Rosa, F.G.; Corcione, S.; Montrucchio, G.; Brazzi, L.; Di Perri, G. Appropriate Treatment of Invasive Candidiasis in ICU: Timing, Colonization Index, Candida Score & Biomarkers, Towards de-Escalation? *Turk. J. Anaesthesiol. Reanim.* **2016**, *44*, 279–282. [CrossRef] [PubMed]
36. Timsit, J.-F.; Bassetti, M.; Cremer, O.; Daikos, G.; De Waele, J.; Kallil, A.; Kipnis, E.; Kollef, M.; Laupland, K.; Paiva, J.-A.; et al. Rationalizing antimicrobial therapy in the ICU: A narrative review. *Intensive Care Med.* **2019**, *45*, 172–189. [CrossRef] [PubMed]
37. Kollef, M.H.; Shorr, A.F.; Bassetti, M.; Timsit, J.-F.; Micek, S.T.; Michelson, A.P.; Garnacho-Montero, J. Timing of antibiotic therapy in the ICU. *Crit. Care* **2021**, *25*, 360. [CrossRef] [PubMed]
38. Tabah, A.; Bassetti, M.; Kollef, M.H.; Zahar, J.-R.; Paiva, J.-A.; Timsit, J.-F.; Roberts, J.A.; Schouten, J.; Giamarellou, H.; Rello, J.; et al. Antimicrobial de-escalation in critically ill patients: A position statement from a task force of the European Society of Intensive Care Medicine (ESICM) and European Society of Clinical Microbiology and Infectious Diseases (ESCMID) Critically Ill Patients Study Group (ESGCIP). *Intensive Care Med.* **2020**, *46*, 245–265. [CrossRef]

MDPI
St. Alban-Anlage 66
4052 Basel
Switzerland
Tel. +41 61 683 77 34
Fax +41 61 302 89 18
www.mdpi.com

Journal of Clinical Medicine Editorial Office
E-mail: jcm@mdpi.com
www.mdpi.com/journal/jcm

www.ingramcontent.com/pod-product-compliance
Lightning Source LLC
Chambersburg PA
CBHW062053220926
51850CB00010B/2752
9783036583808